INSTANT ALLERGY

Instant Allergy

NIELS MYGIND
Associate Professor
Department of Respiratory Diseases
University Hospital of Århus
Denmark

RONALD DAHL
Professor
Department of Respiratory Diseases
University Hospital of Århus
Denmark

SØREN PEDERSEN
Professor
Department of Paediatrics
University Hospital of Odense
Denmark

KRISTIAN THESTRUP-PEDERSEN
Professor
Department of Dermatology
University of Århus
Marselisborg Hospital
Århus, Denmark

b

**Blackwell
Science**

© 1997 by
Blackwell Science Ltd
Editorial Offices:
Osney Mead, Oxford OX2 0EL
25 John Street, London WC1N 2BL
23 Ainslie Place, Edinburgh EH3 6AJ
350 Main Street, Malden
  MA 02148 5018, USA
54 University Street, Carlton
  Victoria 3053, Australia

Other Editorial Offices:
Arnette Blackwell SA
  224, Boulevard Saint Germain
  75007 Paris, France

Blackwell Wissenschafts-Verlag GmbH
Kurfürstendamm 57
10707 Berlin, Germany

Zehetnergasse 6
A-1140 Wien
Austria

First published 1997

Printed and bound in Italy
by Rotolito Lombarda S.p.A., Milan

The Blackwell Science logo is a
trade mark of Blackwell Science Ltd,
registered at the United Kingdom
Trade Marks Registry

DISTRIBUTORS

Marston Book Services Ltd
PO Box 269
Abingdon
Oxon OX14 4YN
(*Orders*: Tel: 01235 465500
            Fax: 01235 465555)

USA
Blackwell Science, Inc.
Commerce Place
350 Main Street,
Malden, MA 02148 5018
(*Orders*: Tel: 800 759 6102
                  617 388 8250
            Fax: 617 388 8255)

Canada
Copp Clark Professional
200 Adelaide Street West, 3rd Floor
Toronto, Ontario M5H 1W7
(*Orders*: Tel: 416 597-1616
                  800 815-9417
            Fax: 416 597-1617)

Australia
Blackwell Science Pty Ltd
54 University Street
Carlton, Victoria 3053
(*Orders*: Tel: 3 9347 0300
            Fax: 3 9347 5001)

A catalogue record for this title
is available from the British Library

ISBN 0-632-04232-X

Library of Congress
Cataloging-in-publication Data

Instant allergy/
Niels Mygind . . . [et al.].
      p.   cm.
  Abbreviated ed. of:
  Essential allergy. 2nd ed. 1996.
  Includes bibliographical references
  and index.
  ISBN 0–632–04232–X
  1 Allergy.   I Mygind, Niels.
  II Essential allergy.
  [DNLM: 1 Hypersensitivity.
  WD 300 I59 1997]
  RC584.I548   1997
  616.97—dc20
  DNLM/DLC
  for Library of Congress   96–44629
                                     CIP

Contents

Preface

Allergic diseases are common and they have increased in frequency over the last decades. More than 30% of the total population today suffer from eczema, hay fever or asthma, which apparently are the diseases of modern society.

Severely allergic patients are treated by specialists in allergy and dermatology, and we have earlier addressed these specialists in the text *Essential Allergy* (Blackwell Science, 1996). However, most of the cases of eczema, hay fever and asthma are mild, and they are often treated by general practitioners and by specialists in fields other than allergy and dermatology.

Instant Allergy is an abbreviated edition of *Essential Allergy*, and it offers these groups of colleagues an updated, practically oriented, and illustrated text on the allergic diseases. 'Instant' refers to an easily understood text which can be read in a weekend (Friday included).

Niels Mygind
Ronald Dahl
Søren Pedersen
Kristian Thestrup-Pedersen

Acronyms and abbreviations

APC	antigen presenting cell
ASA	triad consisting of intolerance to acetylsalicylic acid, nasal polyps/sinusitis and asthma
AU	allergy unit
Bm cell	B memory cell
BU	biological unit
C1-9	complement components 1–9
CD	cluster of differentiation
CFC	chloro-fluoro-carbon (freon)
CNS	central nervous system
COPD	chronic obstructive pulmonary disease
CT	computed tomography
DPI	dry-powder inhaler
ECP	eosinophil cationic protein
FcεR1	high-affinity receptor for IgE
FcεR2	low-affinity receptor for IgE
FESS	functional endoscopic sinus surgery
FEV_1	forced expiratory volume in 1 second
FVC	forced vital capacity
GM-CSF	granulocyte-macrophage colony stimulating factor
HPA	hypothalamic pituitary adrenal
ICAM-1	intercellular adhesion molecule 1
IgE	immunoglobulin E
IL	interleukin
IFN	interferon
kPa	kilopascal
LTB-E	leukotrienes B–E
MC_{CT}	mast cell containing chymase and tryptase (connective tissue mast cell)
MC_T	mast cell containing tryptase (mucosal mast cell)
MBP	major basic protein
MDI	metered-dose inhaler

NSAID	non-steroidal anti-inflammatory drug
$PaCO_2$	arterial blood gas tension of CO_2
PAF	platelet activating factor
PaO_2	arterial blood gas tension of O_2
PEF	peak expiratory flow
PC_{20}	provoking concentration (of histamine) which reduces lung function 20%
PGD-F	prostaglandins D–F
PRIST	paper radioimmunosorbent test
prn	*pro re nata*: as circumstances may require, i.e. when a drug is used on an as-needed basis
RAST	radioallergosorbent test
RIST	radioimmunosorbent test
RV	residual volume
SaO_2	arterial blood gas saturation of O_2
Tc cell	T cytotoxic cell
Th cell	T helper cell
Tm cell	T memory cell
TNF	tumour necrosis factor
VCAM-1	vascular cell adhesion molecule 1
VC	vital capacity
VIP	vasoactive intestinal polypeptide

Chapter 1: The cells and molecules of allergy

You can offer optimal treatment of allergic rhinitis, asthma, urticaria and eczema to your patients without knowing the existence of Langerhans' cells, Th2 lymphocytes, cytokines and high-affinity receptors for IgE. But if you are curious about the recent and spectacular advances in the molecular biology and immunology behind allergic diseases then you can spend a few hours reading the very brief introduction below.

The immune system

Self and non-self. It is the unique ability and the primary aim of the immune system, consisting of lymphocytes and antibody molecules, to *distinguish between 'self' and 'non-self'*, that is between macromolecules, which are products of the individual's own genes, and those which are not.

Specificity. When a non-self macromolecule penetrates into the organism it acts as an *antigen* and stimulates the immune system exclusively towards that molecule, or towards a part of it, an *epitope*.

B and T cells. Lymphocytes which have not been in contact with their antigen are called '*naive cells*'. When naive *B lymphocytes* are stimulated by antigen, they are transformed into *plasma cells* which synthesize *antibody*, and this is called a *humoral immune response* (Fig. 1.1). Antigen stimulation of naive *T lymphocytes* causes them to differentiate into *activated T cells*, which secrete a series of biologically active proteins, cytokines, and that is a *cell-mediated immune response*.

T helper and T cytotoxic cells. *T helper cells* and their signal proteins, the cytokines, control the entire immune response. They play an important role both in IgE synthesis and in recruiting and activating inflammatory cells in the IgE-mediated allergic

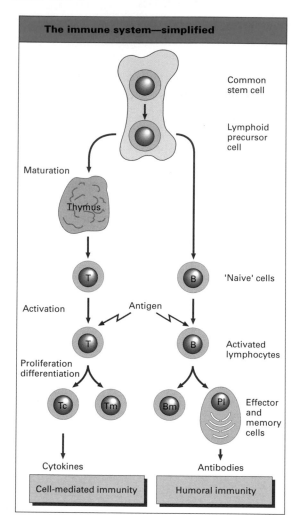

Fig. 1.1 The two lymphocyte subsets, T and B cells, are both derived from precursor cells in the bone marrow. Maturation in the thymus is only needed for the T cells. Antigen stimulation activates the cells, which proliferate and differentiate into memory cells (Tm, Bm) and effector cells. The T cell line operates by effector or cytotoxic T cells (Tc) and the productions of cytokines, while the B cell line operates by the formation of antibodies. Cell-mediated immunity (left arm) and humoral immunity (right arm) are exemplified by the tuberculin reaction and by hay fever, respectively.

reaction. *T cytotoxic cells*, or T effector cells, kill antigen-containing cells by direct contact and by the release of cytokines.

Immune protection and immune disease. The term *hypersensitivity* indicates a specifically increased response, depending upon a reaction between antigen and antibody or sensitized lymphocytes, leading to symptoms and morbidity. For clinical practice, it is useful to make a distinction between *immune protection* (against infection) and *immune disease* (allergy and autoimmune disease).

Definition of allergy. The term *allergy* is used when an antigen, which is not harmful in itself, causes an immune response and reaction, which gives rise to symptoms and disease in a few predisposed individuals only. Most of the allergy discussed in this book is *IgE-mediated allergy*. An antigen which induces an IgE response is called an *allergen*.

Type I–IV hypersensitivity reactions

Antigen stimulation of the immune system results in an integrated immune response involving both antibodies and sensitized lymphocytes. Nevertheless, the simplified classification of Gell and Coombs into four distinct types is convenient.

Type I or IgE-mediated reaction. When allergen reacts with IgE antibody, attached to the surface of a mast cell, the cell degranulates and liberates histamine and other *chemical mediators*. Symptoms occur within minutes, and a Type I reaction is, therefore, an *immediate reaction*. This reaction is followed by eosinophil inflammation, which is caused by the secretion of cytokines from T cells (and from mast cells). *Allergic rhinitis* is an example of a disease based on a Type I reaction

Type II or cytotoxic reaction occurs between cell-bound antigen and circulating IgG or IgM antibody. *Transfusion reactions*, drug-induced *haemolytic anaemia*, thrombocytopenia, and agranulocytosis are examples of Type II reactions.

Type III or immune complex reaction occurs between circulating antigen and IgG antibody, and it can result in vasculitis. Type II and III reactions will not be mentioned further in this book.

Type IV or cell-mediated reaction. The activated T cells react with antigen-containing cells and induce the classical *delayed type hypersensitivity* in which symptoms appear 24–48 hours after antigen exposure. Delayed-type hypersensitivity occurs as a result of persistent microbial infection, and a well known example is the *Mantoux reaction* to tuberculin. Allergic *contact eczema* is another example, described later (see Chapter 8).

Antigen presenting cells

A T lymphocyte cannot recognize antigen in solution. It needs to have it presented by an APC. Macrophages and dendritic or Langerhans' cells are APCs. Most important in skin and airways are the Langerhans' cells. They pick up the antigen, break down the protein molecule into small peptide fragments, recognizable by T lymphocytes, and they travel to the regional lymph nodes to activate the T cells.

Cell receptors

The first step in the immune response is the APC's handling of the antigen. The next step, which is either stimulation of T lymphocytes or the formation of antibodies, requires specific antigen recognition. This is effected by cell receptors, which are protein molecules in the cell membrane through which the cell communicates with the environment. A cell receptor has specificity for another protein molecule, called its *ligand.*

Cell receptors are necessary for the lymphocytes' specific recognition of the antigen. The antigen-recognizing receptor on T cells is called the *T-cell antigen receptor*, and on B cells it is a membrane immunoglobulin molecule.

CD markers. Each cell receptor is given a CD number, which is also used for the identification of different cell types. For example, T cells are named CD3$^+$ cells, because they have the T-cell receptor CD3. B cells are CD20⁺, and T cytotoxic cells CD8⁺. The CD4⁺ T helper cells are best known, because the CD4 marker is, unfortunately, also the receptor for HIV infection.

Cytokines

Cytokines are soluble protein molecules produced by one cell that alter the behaviour or properties of another cell.

Terminology. Some cytokines are referred to as *interleukins* (IL-1 to IL-17), while other cytokines are named *granulocyte-macrophage colony stimulating factor* (GM-CSF), *interferons* (IFN), and *tumour necrosis factor* (TNF).

Role in cell-to-cell communication. In a functional immune system, a number of cells must coordinate their activities, as in the nervous system, and this cell-to-cell communication is effected by the cytokines, acting as *signal proteins*.

A series of cytokine molecules work in collaboration, providing the *cytokine network* fundamental to every function of the immune response and inflammation. In popular terms, each cytokine is a single 'word' in the 'sentence' of instructions given from one cell to another. Cytokines have recently become crucial to the understanding of the mechanisms underlying allergic diseases.

Effects. Cytokines act as haemopoietic growth factors and as chemotactic factors (chemokines), they have regulatory roles in the immune system, and they have pro-inflammatory effects and cytotoxic effects.

Some cytokines are of particular importance in allergy. *IL-3* stimulates the growth of precursors of *eosinophils, basophils* and *mast cells. IL-4* acts on B cells to induce the so-called IgE isotype switching and the *production of IgE antibody. IL-5* is chiefly a growth and differentiation factor for eosinophils, and it also prolongs their survival. IL-5 is, at least in part, responsible for the *eosinophilia* in allergic diseases.

Cytokine-forming cells. The important cytokines in allergic disease are produced by the following: T lymphocytes (of the Th2 subset), mast cells, eosinophils, epithelial cells, and by other cell types as well.

Th1 and Th2 cells

There are two types of Th cells, Th1 and Th2, characterized by their cytokine profile (Fig. 1.2). Th1 cells are preferably stimulated by microbial antigens, and Th2 cells by allergens (and by parasites). *Th1 cells* produce *IL-2* and *IFN-γ*. *Th2 cells* produce *IL-4, IL-5* (IL-10 and IL-13), and both cell types produce IL-3 and GM-CSF.

While the cytokine profile of Th1 cells predominantly leads to delayed-type hypersensitivity and to IgG synthesis, the Th2 cytokines induce the synthesis of IgE and lead to eosinophilia. It is interesting to note that the two systems, by their release of cytokines, are mutually suppressive (Fig. 1.2).

IgE

IgE is produced by B lymphocytes and plasma cells in the airways, gastro-intestinal tract and regional lymph nodes. It occurs in a very low concentration and comprises less than 0.001% of circulating immunoglobulin.

The initial formation of IgE antibody depends upon signals from Th2 lymphocytes and IL-4. As IFN-γ, produced by Th1 cells, can antagonize the process, the ratio between activated Th2 and Th1 cells seems to be a critical factor in IgE regulation.

Receptors for IgE

Injection of IgE antibody can sensitize the skin to allergen for prolonged periods. This *skin-sensitizing* ability of IgE is due to the fact that it binds to *mast cells* and *basophils*, which have *high-affinity receptors* for IgE (FcεR1). There are low-affinity receptors (FcεR2) on other cells (T cells, eosinophils, APCs) but their role in allergic reactions is uncertain. Molecular biologists have now characterized the exact amino acid sequence in both the IgE molecule and in the receptors for IgE.

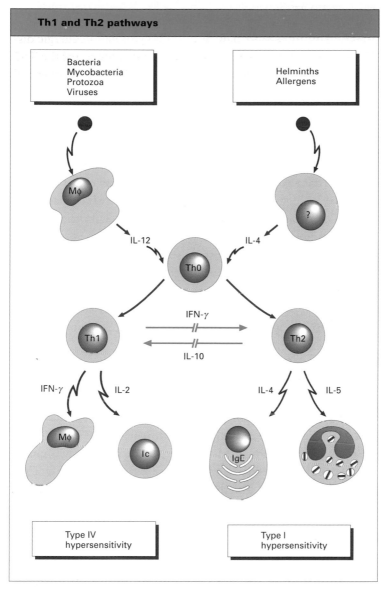

Fig. 1.2 Stimulation with different types of antigen of 'naive' Th0 cells results in the formation of one of two functional Th lymphocyte subsets with different cytokine profiles. Antigens, derived from micro-organisms, stimulate Th1 cells by the release of IL-12 from macrophages, while allergens stimulate Th2 cells by IL-4. Stimulation of Th1 cells results in a cell-mediated, delayed-type hypersensitivity (a Type IV reaction) and in IgG synthesis, while Th2 cells are responsible for humoral immunity and IgE-mediated allergy (a Type I reaction). The two systems are mutually suppressive.

Mast cells and basophils

These cells are the primary initiating cells of IgE-mediated allergic reactions, as they have high-affinity receptors for IgE and synthesize and release histamine and other chemical mediators. They are very important for eliciting symptoms in allergic rhinitis and urticaria, but their role in asthma and atopic dermatitis seems less significant.

Cellular characteristics. The *mast cell* is a tissue cell, predominant in skin, airways and gastro-intestinal tract. It is characterized by *granules*, which contain histamine, leukotrienes and prostaglandins.

There are two types of mast cells: connective tissue mast cells or MC_{TC} (mast cells containing tryptase and chymase) and mucosal mast cells or MC_T (mast cells containing tryptase only). While the MC_{TC} predominate in the skin, it is the MC_T that migrate into the epithelium of the nose and bronchi during allergic reactions.

The *basophil leucocyte* acts as a 'circulating mast cell', which mediates systemic allergic reactions.

Haemopoietic development. Progenitors of mast cells and basophils are formed in the bone marrow under the influence of the cytokines, IL-3 and GM-CSF (Fig. 1.3). The precursor cells are released into the blood and migrate into the tissue. IL-5 is a specific growth and differentiation factor for basophils (and eosinophils).

Degranulation. *Allergen* causes activation and degranulation of the cells by interaction with IgE antibody, bound to the FcεR1 receptor. Another cause of degranulation and mediator release is *non-immunological factors*. The list is long and includes mechanical and thermal trauma, venoms, activation of the complement cascade, some cytokines, drugs (plasma expanders, muscle relaxants, morphine), and radiocontrast media.

Mast cell degranulation not only occurs in allergic disease but

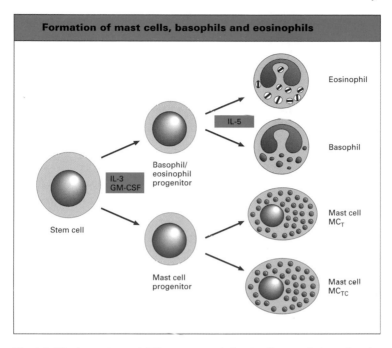

Formation of mast cells, basophils and eosinophils

Fig. 1.3 The formation and differentiation of allergic effector cells is mediated by cytokines which act as haemopoietic growth factors.

also in non-allergic asthma, rhinitis, nasal polyps and urticaria; the nature of the major trigger mechanism is unknown.

Chemical mediators

Chemical mediators, released from mast cells and basophils, are either stored in the *granules* (histamine) or newly synthesized from lipids in the *cell membrane*. Each mediator has many effects in the tissue and the exact role of individual mediators in the pathophysiology of allergic diseases, for example asthma, is not yet clear.

Histamine stimulates nerve endings, contracts smooth muscles and increases vascular permeability. In the *skin*, it induces the typical wheal-and-flare reaction. In the *nose*, it causes itching, hypersecretion and blockage. *Bronchial* histamine inhalation results in bronchoconstriction. High plasma levels can result in *anaphylaxis*. All these effects are mediated through H_1 histamine receptors.

Lipid mediators, or membrane-derived mediators, are the *leukotrienes* (LTB$_4$, LTC$_4$, LTD$_4$ and LTE$_4$) PGD$_2$, thromboxane, and PAF. In contrast to histamine, their formation is not confined to mast cells and basophils. Pertubation of the cell membrane of almost all nucleated cells, including the eosinophil, induces the synthesis of lipid mediators. They are potent mediators, producing smooth-muscle contraction, mucus secretion, and increased vascular permeability. The lipid mediators, LTs in particular, play an important pathogenic role in *asthma*.

Eosinophils

Eosinophil proteins. The eosinophil leucocyte is an important cell in the allergic inflammation. It can easily be identified by its bright red *granules*. They are made up of eosinophil-specific proteins (MBP and ECP). These proteins are *cytotoxic* and contribute to tissue damage, for example, *epithelial shedding in asthma*.

Cell formation. The eosinophil is formed *in the bone marrow* under the control of the cytokine growth factors, *GM-CSF, IL-3, IL-5* (Fig. 1.3), all of which can be produced by Th2 cells.

Adhesion molecules and eosinophilia. The cell circulates in the blood for a few days. It leaves the circulation when *adhesion molecules* are activated (upregulated) in an inflamed tissue (Fig. 1.4). Cellular adhesion molecules, *on endothelial cells and on leucocytes*, play a very important role in physical *cell-to-cell contact*. An adhesion molecule and its ligand (counterpart) make the cells 'sticky' and hold them together as long as it is necessary for their 'communication'.

Adhesion molecules are grouped into the *selectins*, the *immunoglobulin superfamily* (ICAM-1, VCAM-1) and the

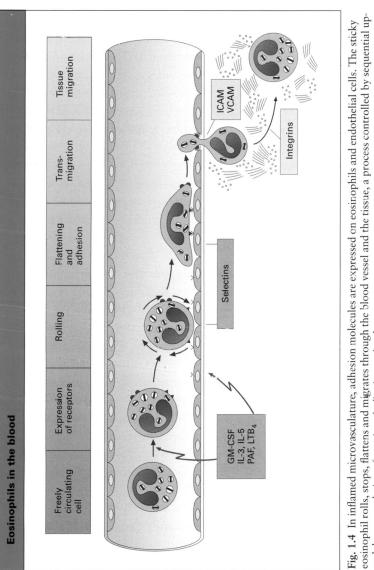

Eosinophils in the blood

Freely circulating cell	Expression of receptors	Rolling	Flattening and adhesion	Trans-migration	Tissue migration

GM-CSF
IL-3, IL-5
PAF, LTB$_4$

Selectins

ICAM
VCAM

Integrins

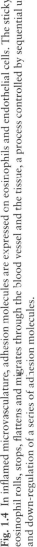

Fig. 1.4 In inflamed microvasculature, adhesion molecules are expressed on eosinophils and endothelial cells. The sticky eosinophil rolls, stops, flattens and migrates through the blood vessel and the tissue, a process controlled by sequential up- and down-regulation of a series of adhesion molecules.

integrins. Cytokines, in inflamed areas, upregulate these adhesion molecules one-by-one. When this happens, the freely circulating eosinophil becomes attached to endothelial cells, rolls slowly along them, flattens (selectins), migrates between the cells (ICAM-1, VCAM-1), and passes through the connective tissue (integrins) by directed migration towards *chemotactic factors.*

In the tissue, *the eosinophil becomes activated* and *secretes its cytotoxic proteins* and also some cell membrane-derived lipid mediators (LTC$_4$, PGE$_2$, PAF). The local survival of eosinophils is considerably prolonged during allergic inflammation (Fig. 1.5).

Allergen challenge

An allergen challenge or provocation test is used as a simple model for studying allergic inflammation and the pathophysiology of allergic diseases. It results in an early and a late response (Fig. 1.6).

The early response starts within minutes and symptoms and signs have usually resolved within an hour. There is evidence of *mast cell degranulation.*

The early response in the *skin* is characterized by itching and a *wheal-and-flare* reaction, almost completely blocked by an H$_1$ antihistamine, which indicates that it is caused by histamine.

The response in the *bronchi* is due to *smooth-muscle contraction,* prevented and reversed by an inhaled beta$_2$ bronchodilator. Antagonists of LTs and of histamine have partial effects.

In the *nose, sneezing, watery rhinorrhoea* and *blockage* can be inhibited by an H$_1$ antihistamine to a high, a moderate and a low degree, respectively. The drug can almost completely inhibit *eye-itching* and *conjunctival redness.*

The late response often develops after 4–6 hours. Predisposing factors are a severe allergen challenge and inflammation in the tissue before the challenge.

During the late response, there is accumulation and activation of *Th2 cells, eosinophils* and other cells, which all, by their release of cytokines, mediators and cytotoxic proteins,

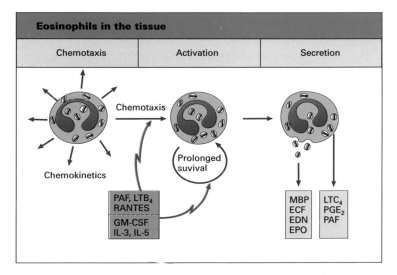

Fig. 1.5 Eosinophils are attracted to inflamed areas by chemotactic substances, they become activated and secrete their cytotoxic proteins and mediators.

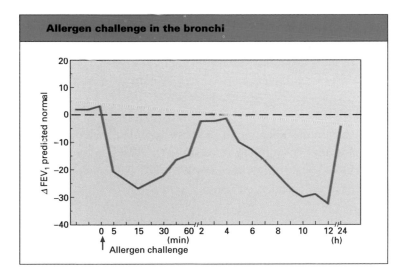

Fig. 1.6 Allergen inhalation challenge can cause an isolated early response, but it often results in a dual response, consisting of an early and a late phase, showing a typical biphasic curve.

contribute to an *inflammatory reaction*. *Corticosteroids* very efficiently block the development of late responses in all tissues.

An early *bronchial* response is usually, but not always, followed by a late response, and measurement of lung function shows a typical *biphasic curve* (Fig. 1.6). The late response is a better *model for chronic asthma disease* than the early response, because it is associated with an increase in bronchial responsiveness. The late symptoms in the *nose* are *mild* and *variable in time*.

Allergic inflammation

Atopic dermatitis. In the skin, there is an increased number of Langerhans' cells, Th2 cells, mast cells and eosinophils.

Asthma. There is: (1) an *increased number of epithelial mast cells* (of the MC_T type), showing signs of degranulation; (2) an increased number of activated *Th2 cells*, which secrete *IL-5* of importance for eosinophil accumulation; (3) upregulation of *adhesion molecules* (ICAM-1) in vasculature and also in surface epithelium; (4) an increased number of *eosinophils*, showing signs of activation and release of their cytotoxic proteins (Fig. 1.7); and (5) *epithelial damage and shedding*, in particular in severe asthma.

Allergic rhinitis. There is an increased number of Langerhans' cells, eosinophils and mast cells of the MC_T type in the epithelium. Histological studies have failed to show any morphological damage to the surface epithelium.

Conjunctivitis. The allergic inflammation is much more pronounced in *vernal kerato-conjunctivitis* than in *allergic conjunctivitis*.

Hyper-responsiveness

It is characteristic of allergic inflammation in all allergic diseases that a series of physical and chemical stimuli, causing little or no reaction in normal subjects, results in sneezing, coughing,

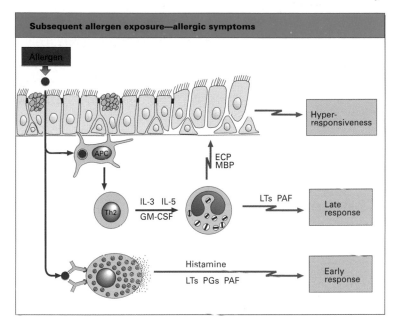

Fig. 1.7 Simplified presentation of the allergic reaction in the airways. The interaction between allergen and mast cells results in the early response, while other cell types are involved in the late response and in the development of hyper-responsiveness.

wheezing, itching and scratching. This *hyper-responsiveness*, or *hyper-reactivity*, is best studied in asthma.

Allergen challenge of the bronchi, showing a late response, will result in an increased bronchial responsiveness, as will natural exposure to allergen.

Eosinophils are the major cause of airway hyper-responsiveness, because their *cytotoxic proteins* (ECP, MBP) damage the epithelial cells so the sensory nerves more easily become exposed to irritants (Fig. 1.7).

Persistent and transient hyper-responsiveness. Patients with *chronic asthma* have a relatively stable degree of airway hyper-responsiveness. Superimposed on this persistent baseline responsiveness, transient increases develop following exposure to allergens, chemical sensitizers, noxious gases and viral respiratory tract infections.

Chapter 2: Allergy: an increasing problem

Atopic diseases

Atopy refers to a hereditary predisposition to produce IgE antibody. When *atopic subjects* are exposed to the minute amounts of protein allergens in the environment, they respond with a persistent production of IgE antibody. The *atopic status* of a person can be determined by skin-testing with a battery of common allergens. The most important *atopic diseases* are atopic dermatitis, allergic rhinitis and asthma.

While allergic rhinitis and asthma are *IgE-mediated* diseases, atopic dermatitis is, in most cases, merely *IgE-associated.* In other words, allergic rhinitis and asthma are *atopic and allergic diseases* in which symptoms are the result of allergen exposure, while atopic dermatitis is an *atopic disease but not an allergic disease,* for symptoms are not, or are only to a minor degree, caused by allergen exposure. When atopic dermatitis is called allergic it results in futile attempts to find an offending allergen.

A *highly atopic patient* develops atopic dermatitis, allergic rhinitis and asthma in childhood. The patient is an 'allergy machine' and he easily becomes sensitized to new allergens. A patient who merely develops pollen allergy in adolescence usually has a *low degree of atopy*, and the risk of further sensitization and development of other atopic manifestations is low. Fortunately, this example is by far the most frequent.

Occurrence of atopic diseases

A *positive skin test* to allergens occurs in *20–30%* of the total population and *15–20%* will develop an *atopic disease* (mild cases included). The highest prevalence rate is reached at *15–30 years of age* (Fig. 2.1). Once developed, a positive skin test will not disappear although the symptoms, of hay fever for example, may have ceased.

Development of atopic diseases

The development of atopic allergic disease depends upon: (1) *genetic predisposition*; (2) *exposure to allergens*; and perhaps (3) exposure to 'adjuvants' which may facilitate the sensitization process.

Genetic factors. The risk for the child is doubled when one parent is atopic and quadrupled when both are atopic. A child inherits a predisposition for (1) *atopic disease in general*; (2) involvement of *certain organs*; and (3) *severity* of the disease. A child of parents with severe eczema and asthma is therefore at greater risk than a child of parents with simple hay fever.

Exposure to food allergens. An early introduction of potential allergens in infant feeding is associated with an increased risk of atopic disease. This may not be surprising, as mother's milk is the natural food for babies and cow's milk for cattle. Exclusive breast-feeding can reduce the prevalence rate of *gastro-intestinal allergy symptoms* and of *atopic dermatitis*.

Exposure to aero-allergens is *the primary cause of the development of asthma in children* and young adults. Children who have been exposed to high levels of mite antigen have a *5–10-fold increased risk* of mite sensitization and asthma. Also, other allergens, derived from cats, dogs, cockroaches and moulds, are capable of increasing the prevalence of allergy and asthma. It is the prophylactic implications that early *allergen avoidance regimens can prevent the onset of asthma*, and of allergic rhinitis, in a considerable number of susceptible infants.

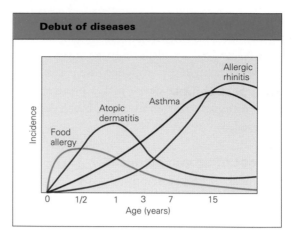

Fig. 2.1 Approximate incidence (first appearance of symptoms) of atopic diseases in relation to age.

Month of birth. Babies born in the months immediately before a pollen season have a somewhat increased risk of developing pollen allergy later in life. This observation has no practical clinical consequence, but it shows that the first few months of life, when the immune system is immature, is an immunologically vulnerable period.

Parental smoking and air pollution. It has been speculated that some factors, acting as 'adjuvants', can facilitate the sensitization process and increase the occurrence of allergic diseases. While parental smoking, indoor gas-heating and outdoor air pollution can increase the occurrence of wheezy illness in children and induce wheezing in all asthmatics, it is dubious whether these factors can facilitate the sensitization process. Epidemiological studies have not supported the claim that air pollution is an important adjuvant.

Rural and urban areas. There is a somewhat higher prevalence rate of atopic diseases in urban than in rural areas.

Western style of living. The prevalence of atopic disease increases when people move to industrialized countries, changing from native to a western lifestyle and living conditions.

Increasing prevalence

The cause is unknown. The prevalence of atopic dermatitis, allergic rhinitis and asthma has increased in western countries since World War II (Fig. 2.2; Table 2.1). Increased awareness of allergic diseases can only be part of the explanation, which must be sought in *environmental factors.*

The reduced practice of breast-feeding and the early introduction of cow's milk to infants in modern societies may explain some of the increase in atopic dermatitis.

The quantity of *aero-allergens* has not increased in general. However, *increased mite exposure* occurs when energy-saving homes with little ventilation and high humidity are built in

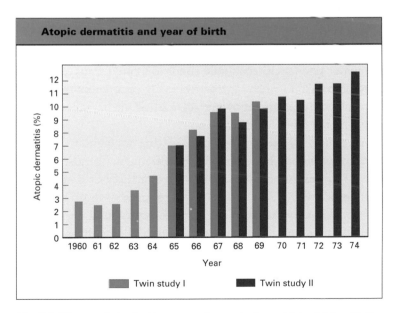

Fig. 2.2 The cumulative incidence rates for atopic dermatitis in children (0–7 years) according to year of birth. (From Schultz Larsen F, Hanifin JM. Secular change in the occurrence of atopic dermatitis. *Acta Derm Venereol (Stockh),* 1992; suppl **176**: 7–12.)

Increasing prevalence of disease		
	Prevalence (%)	
	1971	1981
Allergic rhinitis	4.4	8.4
Asthma	1.9	2.8

Table 2.1 Prevalence of allergic rhinitis and asthma in young Swedish men. (From Åberg N. Asthma and allergic rhinitis in Swedish conscripts. *Clin Exp Allergy*, 1989; 19: 59–63.)

temperate zones and when people indigenous to tropical climates change their sleeping habits by the use of blankets.

As mentioned above, it is doubtful whether *air pollution* plays any role in the allergic sensitization process, but this is frequently claimed.

It is highly unsatisfactory that the main reason for the increasing prevalence of atopic disease remains *unknown*.

A sign of health? A nutritionally compromised population, living under poor socio-economic conditions, frequently develops chronic recurrent infections which easily become invasive, for example, mastoiditis following acute otitis media. Allergic diseases, on the other hand, are rare.

An affluent western population, getting adequate food, proteins, vitamins and minerals, has a low frequency of severe invasive infections, but the prevalence of atopic diseases is high.

Recent research has suggested the existence of a Yin–Yang relationship between infection (Th1 cell cytokines) and allergy (Th2 cell cytokines). If allergy is a sign of wealth and health, prevention will be difficult!

Prediction and prevention

When the start of a prevention programme is indicated, the patient's parents should be informed that even the best avoidance programme can only reduce and not eliminate the risk of atopic disease (Table 2.2).

Preventive programme and occurrence of disease		
	Occurrence (%)	
	With preventive programme	Without programme
Atopic dermatitis	14	31
Vomiting/diarrhoea	5	20
Colic	9	24
Cow's milk allergy	5	20

Table 2.2 Occurrence of atopic dermatitis and food allergy at age 18 months in high-risk infants with and without a preventive programme (see Table 2.3). (From Halken S, Høst A, Hansen LG, Østerballe O. Effect of an allergy prevention programme on incidence of atopic symptoms in infancy. *Allergy*, 1992; 47: 545–53.)

Identify high-risk babies. Stringent prevention programmes are expensive and can easily cause significant disturbance in family life. They are advised for *high-risk babies (fetus)* who have *both parents with atopic disease* or *one with severe disease*.

Time period for intervention. As described above, the first months of life are the most important for allergic sensitization and it is usually advised to carry out prevention programmes for at least 4–6 months.

Preventive diet. *Maternal dieting cannot be recommended.* It is without proven efficacy and pregnant women and lactating mothers need good nutrition. Breast-feeding provides protection against the development of atopic dermatitis and food allergy. *Strict breast-feeding for 4–6 months* and delayed introduction of solid food is recommended for high-risk babies (Table 2.3). When necessary, breast-milk can be supplemented by a hypo-allergenic formula, although this is expensive.

Avoidance of aero-allergens. The intervention programme is best started before the child is born. The bedroom is made as clean and 'mite-hostile' as possible (see Table 18.1). Furred pets

Prevention of allergy in high-risk babies
Breast-feeding, at least for 4–6 months, but preferably as long as possible
Avoidance of cow's milk in the maternity unit before breast-feeding is started ('the hidden bottle')
Hypo-allergenic formula as a substitute for breast-feeding when this is needed for nutrition during the first 4–6 months
Complete avoidance of cow's milk during the first 4–6 months
Late and step-wise introduction of solid food
No smoking in the home
No furred pets in the home
Mite avoidance programme in the child's bedroom before birth

Table 2.3 Preventive programme recommended for high-risk babies.

should be removed months before birth as allergen can remain in the furniture for prolonged periods.

Avoidance of smoking. There should be no exposure to tobacco smoke in the home, and smoking parents should be told that their habit will more than double the risk of development of a wheezy illness in their child.

Non-atopic diseases

Atopic allergy is the cause of perennial rhinitis and asthma in 90% of children but only in 30% of adults. Thus, many patients with diseases discussed in this book are not allergic. Chronic urticaria and nasal polyposis are, as a rule, non-allergic.

The cause of these 'allergy-like diseases' is unknown. It is characteristic that they can be associated with *intolerance to acetylsalicylic acid* (aspirin). In such patients, ingestion of acetylsalicylic acid can cause profuse rhinorrhoea, violent asthma, urticaria, angioedema and anaphylactic shock.

The term 'intolerance' is used instead of allergy, as the adverse reaction is *not based on an immune response*. Patients who are intolerant to acetylsalicylic acid will invariably react to other NSAIDs, but they can tolerate paracetamol. Typically, it is part of the so-called ASA triad which consists of: (1) *intolerance to acetylsalicylic acid*; (2) *nasal polyps/hyperplastic sinusitis*; and

(3) *non-allergic asthma*. The full expression of the ASA triad usually develops in *middle-aged patients*, and intolerance to acetylsalicylic acid is very rare in children.

The diagnosis of NSAID intolerance is based on the patient history and, in selected cases, on oral provocation testing. Management consists of strict and life-long avoidance.

Chapter 3: Allergens: the causes of allergy

Characteristics

Antigens that initiate and elicit an IgE-mediated allergic reaction are called *allergens*. Analysis of allergen extracts (e.g. from pollens and mites) has revealed a large number of allergen molecules. Some of these molecules only sensitize a few patients (minor allergens) while others, *major allergens*, evoke an IgE response in most patients.

An allergen molecule consists of a number of *epitopes* (antigenic determinants), which are small polypeptide pieces in the large protein molecule. Patients vary in response both to different allergens and to different epitopes in the same allergen molecule. Different allergens may have some similarities in the amino acid sequence, which result in *cross-reactivity* (e.g. between different grasses).

Determination

It can be *clinically useful* to quantitate environmental allergens. Airborne *pollens* can be sampled in a pollen trap, identified and counted (Fig. 3.1). Immunochemical methods can be used to quantitate *mite* and *animal* allergens in dust collected by a vacuum cleaner. Airborne *mould* spores, sedimented and allowed to grow on culture plates, placed inside a house, can be quantitated by colony counting.

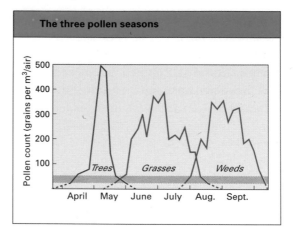

Fig. 3.1 Example of pollen count with a tree season in the spring, a grass season in the summer and a weed (ragweed) season in the early autumn.

Pollen

A pollen grain is released from one plant and transferred to another by insects or by wind. *Insect-pollinated* plants, which attract insects by their colourful flowers, produce few pollens, and only close contact will result in allergy. Most dangerous are the *wind-pollinated* plants which release huge numbers of pollens.

Pollen grains, as relatively large particles (20–30 μm) (Fig. 3.2), are *trapped in the upper airways*, causing rhinitis. Some patients also develop asthma, because allergens, released from pollens in dew and rain drops, as *small dust particles*, can reach the bronchi.

Trees. Many deciduous trees are allergen producers. Pollination usually takes place in the *spring* and is of short duration (see Fig. 3.1). *Birch* is an important cause of allergy in northern parts of Europe, Asia and North America. It cross-reacts with hazel pollen and nut. The *olive tree* is a major cause of pollen allergy in Mediterranean countries. *Japanese cedar* is the most frequent cause of hay fever in Japan.

Grass. Worldwide, grass is the most common cause of pollinosis. There is *extensive cross-reactivity* between most grass species (timothy, rye grass, orchard grass, etc.), so the number of extracts necessary for diagnosis and treatment can be limited to one or a few. Bermuda grass, however, does not cross-react with the above species.

Considerable amounts of pollen are released from *wild and cultivated grass* (hay), and the wind conditions have a profound effect on pollen release and distribution. In the northern hemisphere, the pollen season is later in the north than in the south (important for the planning of summer holidays).

Weeds. *Ragweeds* are the most significant source of allergy in North America, while these plants are rare in Europe. Ragweeds are prominent along roads, at construction sites, on spoil heaps, and, in particular, *in grain fields*. Consequently, cultivated areas (the Midwest in the USA) pose the greatest risk to ragweed-sensitive subjects. The ragweed plants shed pollen in *late summer to*

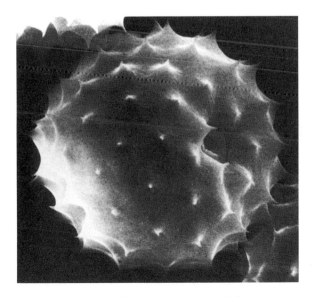

Fig. 3.2 A pollen grain (20 µm) from the giant ragweed plant seen in the scanning electron microscope.

early autumn. The ragweed season occurs later in more southerly areas (in contrast to grass pollen).

Mugwort is of some significance in Europe. *Parietaria* is a common weed and an important allergen source around the Mediterranean basin. It releases pollen almost all year round.

Moulds

Moulds (microfungi) are microscopic plants which depend on plant or animal material for nourishment. Moulds produce vast numbers of small spores (2–5 μm), which reach the lower airways, and *asthma* is therefore the main disease. *Cladosporium, Alternaria, Aspergillus, Penicillium and Mucor* (Fig. 3.3) are causes of mould allergy, which is more important in *children* than in adults.

A *high relative humidity* is essential for growth, and *wet weather favours mould growth.* In warm, humid climates, moulds are present in vast quantities all year round. In temperate zones, spore counts are highest during *late summer.*

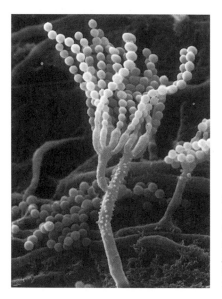

Fig. 3.3 Mould with spores (*Penicillium roqueforti*) seen in the scanning electron microscope. (From Gravesen S, Frisvad JC, Samson RA. *Microfungi.* Copenhagen: Munksgaard, 1994: 1–168.)

Indoors, spores are derived from outside and from *internal growth foci*. Humidity is the determining factor for growth, which can be immense in badly constructed houses ('sick house syndrome'). Moulds can efficiently be disseminated in a building when they grow in the humidifier of an air-conditioning system.

Inhalation of small amounts of allergen in mould spores can evoke an *IgE response* and cause *asthma*. Massive exposure to saprophytic moulds growing in the airway can evoke *IgE and IgG responses* in *bronchopulmonary aspergillosis*. The inhalation of large amounts of mould antigen in organic dust can cause an *IgG response* and *extrinsic allergic alveolitis*.

House dust mites

These mites, not noticeable with the naked eye (Figs 3.4 and 3.5), are the most important source of indoor allergens, and they are the chief cause of '*house dust allergy*'. *Dermatophagoides pteronyssinus* and *D. farinae*, showing strong cross-reactivity, are the most important species.

Requirements. The mites are *vulnerable to desiccation* and usually die when the relative humidity in the surrounding air is below 55%. It is, however, the humidity within their living places that is relevant. Their favourite place is the human bed, where they find all their requirements, i.e. food (the mites *feed from human skin scales*), high humidity and temperature.

Occurrence. The highest concentration of mites is found in dust from the bed, especially from *feather pillows, eiderdowns*, and *old mattresses*. But mites can also thrive in *stuffed furniture, carpets*, and even in *teddy bears*.

Indoor humidity. This varies with the degree of *ventilation* of the rooms and depends upon the *building construction*. The design of western homes in the last 20 years, particularly the manufacture of *airtight, energy-efficient houses*, has led to significant increases in mite levels by reducing ventilation and increasing indoor humidity.

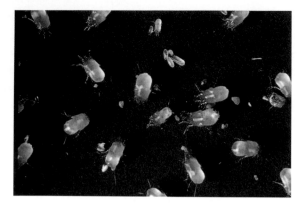

Fig. 3.4 House dust mites alive seen in a stereo microscope. (By courtesy of Matthews J Colloff, Scottish Parasite Diagnostic Laboratory, Stobhill Hospital, Glasgow.)

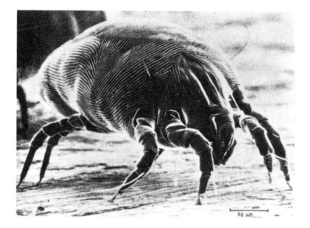

Fig. 3.5 A house dust mite enlarged. Its natural size is 0.3 mm. (From Wharton CW. Mite and commercial extracts of house dust. *Science* 1970; **167**: 1382–5.)

Geographic variation. House dust mites grow best in *warm areas with high humidity* (the tropics). The only areas that appear to be relatively spared of mite contamination are those with a *very dry climate* or those at *high altitudes* (> 3000 metres elevation) (Fig. 3.6).

Seasonal changes. In temperate climates the number of mites is *lowest in the winter* when artificial heating dries out the indoor air. In the tropics, the mite population will *increase following the rainy season*.

Airborne allergen. The mites produce *faeces pellets*, which are the cause of airway symptoms. They are relatively large particles (like pollen grains), and as soon as 30 minutes after disturbance (making the bed, vacuum-cleaning) no, or very little, allergen is airborne. Major *exposure takes place at night* when we have our heads close to mite-infested material. As exposure occurs with closed eyes, conjunctivitis is not a problem.

Storage mites

These mites are known pests of stored *foodstuff* in granaries, warehouses, and food and farm stores. They require a *very high humidity* (rooms with obvious dampness) and are even more sensitive to desiccation than the house dust mites.

A huge number of storage mites, *in stored hay and grain*, is a frequent cause of allergy in farmers. Storage mites are more fre-

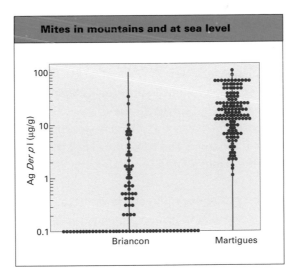

Fig. 3.6 Amounts of mite allergen (*Der p* I) on mattresses at high altitude (Briacon) and at sea level (Martigues). (From Charpin D, Birnbaum J, Haddi E *et al*. Altitude and allergy to house dust mites. *Am Rev Respir Dis*, 1991; **143**: 983–6.)

quent than house dust mites *in tropical dwellings* and are important causes of asthma and rhinitis.

Storage mites do not cross-react with the *Dermatophagoides*
species, and extracts of storage mites *(Glycophagus, Tyropha-
gus, Acarus)* are therefore necessary for an adequate allergy
investigation in some parts of the world.

Cockroaches

Cockroaches are important allergens in *urban dwellings*,
especially in *lower socio-economic communities*. In some inner
city areas (e.g. Chicago, Washington, Atlanta, New York), a
high proportion of asthma and rhinitis patients show a positive
skin test to cockroach extract.

Mammals

Cats and dogs. Allergy to cat and dog proteins is a frequent cause
of symptoms in patients with rhino-conjunctivitis and asthma. In
North America and northern Europe more than half of all homes
have at least one cat or dog.

The major cat allergen is produced predominantly in *salivary
glands*. In dogs, major allergens have been identified in saliva,
epidermal scales (epidermals, dander) and in urine. Hair, as
such, is not allergenic.

Cat allergen is continuously airborne as small particles, and
allergic patients often experience rapid onset of symptoms on
entering a house with a cat. Cat allergens are sticky and become
attached to walls, carpets and furniture. They remain in a home
for months after removal of the animal.

Rodents. Mice, rats, guinea-pigs and hamsters are widely used in
medical research and have gained popularity as *pets*. Their urine
is a potent allergen source. Symptoms usually develop within the
first year of exposure and atopic subjects, especially those allergic to other mammals, have an increased risk of developing allergy.

Horses and cows. Allergy to horses is less of a problem than in
history. The cross-reactivity between *horse dander and serum*

(tetanus vaccine) should be kept in mind. Allergy to cows is mainly a problem for farmers, veterinarians and cowboys. Fortunately, *cow dander* allergic patients tolerate beef-eating.

Birds

It is now realized that the allergenicity of feather extracts, formerly used for skin-testing and injection therapy, is due mainly to contamination with mites. Allergy to *bird-droppings* occurs in individuals having close contact with *pigeons* and *budgerigars* in poorly ventilated rooms. An IgE antibody response results in *asthma*, while an IgG antibody response to bird antigens is a cause of *extrinsic allergic alveolitis*.

Occupational sensitizing agents

Occupational asthma is induced by a *sensitizing agent* inhaled at work. Patients with pre-existing asthma may develop bronchoconstriction at work after exposure to *irritants*.

Prevalence. The introduction of highly reactive chemicals in the manufacture of synthetic materials (plastics) has *increased* the prevalence of occupational asthma over the last few decades, and now represents 5% of adult-onset asthma. In some industries, sensitization develops in as many as 20% of those exposed (Table 3.1).

Types of agents and reactions. The causes of asthma in the workplace can be classified by: (1) the molecular weight of the agents; and (2) the pathogenic response they elicit (Table 3.2). *High molecular weight proteins* act as *allergens* inducing an IgE-mediated reaction. *Low molecular weight chemicals* can act as *haptens* (formation of IgE antibody towards a complex of hapten and human protein), or by a non-IgE-dependent mechanism.

Predisposing factors. These are: heavy *exposure* to molecules having a high sensitizing potency; a high *atopic status; bronchial hyper-responsiveness;* and smoking.

Risk of occupational sensitization	
Sensitizing agent	Frequency (%)
Laboratory animals Enzymes	≥20
Platinum salts Prawn and crab processing	10–20
Acid anhydrides Flour	5–10
Isocyanate Western red cedar	3–5

Table 3.1 Frequency of sensitization to occupational sensitizers among exposed workers.

Occupational sensitizers and pathogenic mechanisms
Allergen and IgE-mediated reaction
Laboratory animals, fish, crustaceans, enzymes, flour, bean dust, gums
Hapten and IgE-mediated reaction
Acid anhydrides, platinum salt, penicillin
Non-IgE-mediated reaction
Grain dust, cotton dust, isocyanates, colophony, Western red cedar

Table 3.2 Sensitizing agents and the reactions by which they induce occupational asthma.

Diagnosis. In the *case history*, the relationship of symptoms to days at work, weekends and holidays is important. Some workers have a classical *immediate reaction* within minutes of coming to work. A *late asthmatic reaction* is common, however. It typically starts 4–8 hours after arrival at work but there is *great variability*, which makes it difficult to draw conclusions based on symptom variation within a 24-hour period.

Usually *symptoms improve during the weekend* but in chronic cases *improvement is only significant during holidays* and workers with severe occupational asthma may deteriorate to such a state that their *airway obstruction may appear fixed*. Such patterns are particularly common in workers exposed to isocyanates and to wood dust.

The history needs objective confirmation from *serial peak flow recordings* at work and at home. Self-recording requires patient compliance and honesty.

Skin-testing and RAST are helpful in diagnosing allergy to proteins and to platinum salts.

Bronchial challenge or exposure-testing are needed for the diagnosis of sensitization to *low molecular weight sensitizers*. The principle of the test is to expose the individual to the putative cause of his asthma in circumstances that resemble, as closely as possible, the conditions of his exposure at work. Challenge with chemicals usually induces both an early and a late response, and testing is time-consuming and potentially hazardous.

Laboratory animals. Workers exposed to *rats, mice* and *guinea-pigs* often develop allergic conjunctivitis, rhinitis and asthma (see above).

Fish and crustaceans. During boiling of *fish, crab* and *prawn*, a vapour is released that often results in sensitization of workers in fisheries.

Enzymes, added to *washing powders*, may sensitize workers in the detergent industry. The consumers are not at risk as the enzymes are added in a granulated or capsulated form that yields little dust.

Grain dust and organic dust. A massive load of organic dust in grain workers and pig-breeders can cause asthma and irre-versibly reduced lung function.

Moulds. Occupational exposure to moulds can occur during manufacture of bread, cheese, beer and wine. In recent years the use of moulds has been extended to include antibiotic, enzyme and steroid manufacture.

Flour. Rhinitis and asthma are common in millers and bakers: *baker's asthma*. The symptoms are usually due to *allergy to* *wheat flour*, but there is considerable cross-reactivity between wheat, rye and barley proteins.

Bean dust. Exposure to dust from *green coffee, castor and soya beans* can cause allergy and asthma.

Cotton dust. Asthma in workers in the cotton industry can be due to inhalation of some concomitant of cotton dust.

Isocyanates. Isocyanates, predominantly *toluene diisocyanate*, are widely used in the manufacture of plastics and other synthetic materials. About 5% of polyurethane foam makers, spray painters and plastic workers develop isocyanate-induced asthma. Symptoms and pathology resemble those of atopic allergic asthma, but the pathogenesis is probably non-allergic, and atopy is not a predisposing factor. The diagnosis is based upon history, identification of isocyanate in the workplace, and a bronchial challenge/exposure test.

Acid anhydrides (trimellitic anhydride, phthalic acid anhydride and others) are widely used as hardening agents in the manufacture of *epoxy resins*, which have a wide range of applications (plastics, adhesives, surface coatings, paints, encapsulation). Workers sensitive to fumes of acid anhydrides have *IgE antibodies* to anhydride–human protein conjugates. Anhydrides have potent *irritant effects* and it may be difficult to distinguish irritant from allergic symptoms.

Wood dust. Sawmill workers can develop asthma due to a *chemical* (plicatic acid) in *hardwoods*, especially *Western red cedar*.
 A diagnosis of red cedar asthma is based on a bronchial challenge test with plicatic acid. It will commonly result in a late bronchial response, and exposed workers often develop *asthma during the night*. The pathogenic mechanism of red cedar asthma is unsolved but bronchial *hyper-responsiveness induced by plicatic acid* seems to play a role.

Colophony. Fumes of the *pine resin*, colophony, when used for soldering or as a glue, is a cause of asthma in workers in the *electrical trades*.

Platinum salts are potent inducers of asthma among *photographic workers* and workers in *metal refineries*. *Positive skin tests*, showing an allergic mechanism, are common and platinum salts can be used directly as skin-test reagents. Asthma can also occur in workers exposed to fumes of salts of nickel, chromium and vanadium.

Non-sensitizing agents. There are many *irritants* in workplaces (sulphur dioxide, nitrogen dioxide, ozone, ammonia, halogen gases), and they induce episodes of asthma in those with bronchial hyper-responsiveness. Typically, asthma occurs *within minutes* and resolves within 1–2 hours of avoidance of exposure. In bronchial inhalation testing, the non-specific irritants provoke an immediate but *not a late response*.

Management and prognosis
When workers are removed from exposure, bronchial hyper-responsiveness is reduced and asthma usually improves. However, following long-lasting exposure, in particular to low molecular weight chemicals (isocyanates, anhydrides, plicatic acid), *asthma may persist* for several years, if not indefinitely. These observations emphasize the importance of *early diagnosis* and *early removal from exposure*.

Chapter 4: Diagnosis of allergy

Skin-testing

This is clinically the most useful allergy test. When the allergen, introduced to the skin, interacts with mast-cell-bound IgE, it induces a *wheal-and-flare reaction* (oedema and erythema) similar to a mosquito bite. Two methods can be used, prick-testing and intracutaneous testing. The prick technique is preferred for clinical routine, but if potent extracts are not available, the more sensitive intracutaneous test can be used.

Prick test. A drop of *glycerinated extract* is placed on the skin, which is punctured by a 1 mm lancet: *prick-puncture test* (Fig. 4.1). The test is simple, quick and virtually painless, it has a high degree of specificity, and the risk of anaphylactic reaction is extremely low. The precision of the test can be improved when it is done *in duplicate*.

Intracutaneous (intradermal) test. An *aqueous extract* from a syringe is injected superficially into the skin. The extracts used are 1000–10 000 times weaker than those used for prick-testing.

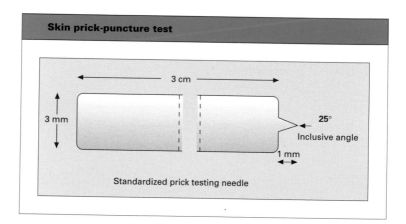

Fig. 4.1 Needle for prick-puncture test. This technique requires little operator skill and gives reproducible results.

The test is highly sensitive but it can induce irritant reactions. Intracutaneous testing is used more in the USA than in Europe.

Controls. A *negative* control with the *diluent* is employed as patients with sensitive (dermographic) skin react to the trauma itself. A *positive* control with *histamine* is used to judge the reactivity of the skin and to discover interfering antihistamine medication.

Allergen extract. It is advisable to use extracts *standardized* by biological testing and by immunochemical methods as they have a consistent potency. The strength of the extract is given in *biological units* (BU/ml) or in *allergy units* (AU/ml).

Factors influencing skin reactivity. *Antihistamines* depress skin reactivity considerably and treatment must be discontinued before testing (4 days are sufficient for most preparations but 4 weeks are needed for astemizole). Systemic steroids, given in anti-asthma dosages, have little effect on the immediate skin reaction, but it is significantly reduced by topical steroid ointments.

Reading the skin reaction. The histamine reaction is maximal after 10 minutes and the allergen reaction after 15 minutes. A positive reaction is suggested by itching and erythema and confirmed by the typical mosquito bite-like, flat elevation (wheal) which is both seen and felt. The largest diameter (D) and the diameter at right angles to this (d) are measured and the reaction is expressed as $D/2 + d/2$. To obtain a permanent record, the wheal can be outlined by a felt-tipped pen and the markings transferred to squared paper by means of tape (Fig. 4.2).

Significance of a positive test. A prick-test wheal of 3 mm or larger is *immunologically specific*, provided the extract is free from irritants (negative reaction in normal subjects).

A positive skin test can occur in a symptom-free subject, *latent allergy*, but a positive pollen test, for instance, indicates a 10-fold

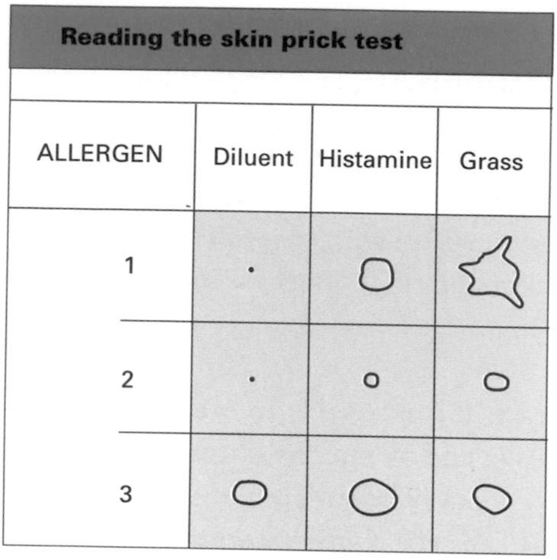

Reading the skin prick test			
ALLERGEN	Diluent	Histamine	Grass
1	.	⭕	🔶
2	.	○	○
3	⭕	⭕	⭕

Fig. 4.2 Examples of a positive skin test to grass pollen (1), a false-negative skin test due to use of antihistamine (2) and a false-positive skin test in a patient with dermographism (3).

increase in the risk of developing hay fever. For a symptomatic patient, exposure to an allergen causing a positive skin test will usually be of *clinical significance*, but a skin test can remain positive years after cessation of symptoms.

While the correlation between a positive skin test and allergen-induced symptoms is good for aero-allergens, it is less good for *food allergens*. Only a fraction of patients with positive tests will react during a food challenge, so *false-positive* reactions are frequent.

Measurement of specific IgE antibody

The radioallergosorbent test (RAST) was the first laboratory test for the detection of *allergen-specific IgE antibody* in serum. While *in vivo* tests measure IgE antibody, mast cell releasability of mediators, and tissue reaction to the mediators, *RAST measures circulating IgE antibody and nothing else*.

While the classical RAST was a specific test with a relatively low sensitivity, a new and improved version (the Pharmacia CAP System) has both high specificity and increased sensitivity.

The *advantages* of RAST include safety, a high degree of precision and standardization, lack of dependence on skin reactivity and medication. The *disadvantages* include lack of immediately available results and high cost.

RAST is mainly used as a supplement to skin-testing when there is doubt regarding the clinical significance of the result, and when a confirmatory test is needed, for example before immunotherapy.

Allergen provocation test

An allergen provocation or challenge test of bronchi, nose and eye is useful for the study of pathophysiology and pharmacodynamics, but it is rarely used for clinical diagnosis.

A bronchial challenge test can be clinically useful for diagnosing allergy to haptens which cannot be used for skin-testing and RAST, but it is tedious and observation for 12 hours is necessary. Controlled inhalation exposure testing can also be of diagnostic value in occupational asthma.

Total serum IgE

IgE, produced in the lymphoid tissue adjacent to the respiratory and gastro-intestinal tracts, eventually becomes *homogeneously distributed* in body fluids and can be measured in the serum. In hay fever, 25–50% of the total IgE is made up of IgE antibody to pollen. Patients with atopic dermatitis often have elevated serum IgE although IgE antibodies, of significance for their skin symptoms, cannot be identified.

Laboratory methods. As the serum IgE level is very low, sensitive immunoassays are required. The first test was the RIST which has now been replaced by the more sensitive and precise *Pharmacia CAP System*.

Normal values. Normal values vary with age (Fig. 4.3). Maternal IgE does not cross the placenta, and the rise in serum IgE is slow during the first year of life. A maximum value is reached in adolescence and it decreases in old age. Characteristically, there

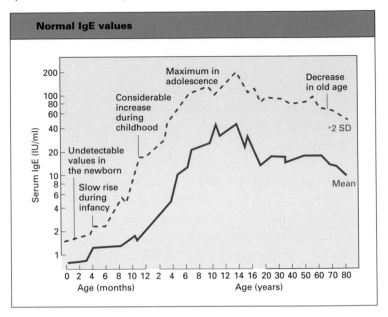

Fig. 4.3 Normal values for total serum IgE. Geometric mean (continuous line) +2 SD (dotted line).

is a wide range for normal values and a considerable overlap between non-atopic and atopic subjects.

IgE in disease. Measurement of total serum IgE is routine in many allergy clinics, but this practice can be questioned by the cost-conscious physician. It is a *valuable* examination when used with care *in selected cases* of atopic dermatitis, allergic rhinitis and asthma. Other diseases with elevated serum IgE are *worm infestations* and *allergic bronchopulmonary aspergillosis*.

Blood eosinophil count

The degree of eosinophilia in blood gives information regarding the *size of the diseased organ*. When the latter is large (lungs, skin), the call-up of eosinophils from the bone marrow is considerable. Consequently, more asthmatic than rhinitis patients have blood eosinophilia (Fig. 4.4).

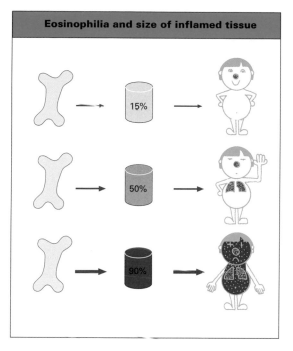

Fig. 4.4 The number of eosinophils transported from the bone marrow to the shock organ depends on its size. Therefore, blood eosinophilia is present in few rhinitis patients, half the asthma patients and the majority of patients with rhinitis, asthma and atopic dermatitis.

In asthma, eosinophilia is related to the disease as such and not to the presence of an IgE-mediated mechanism. The eosinophil count is generally higher in non-allergic than in allergic asthma (Fig. 4.5). There is a positive correlation between the *severity of asthma* and the number of blood eosinophils, so the eosinophil count is a useful guideline for the treatment of the disease, particularly the *requirement for steroids*. Serum measurement of the ECP, which is a marker of eosinophil activation, can give added information. The eosinopenic effect of *corticosteroid* treatment is pronounced and can mask an eosinophilia.

Blood eosinophilia also occurs in worm infestation, Hodgkin's disease, periarteritis nodosa, Löffler's syndrome, hypereosinophilic syndrome, a series of skin diseases, drug allergy, and bronchopulmonary aspergillosis.

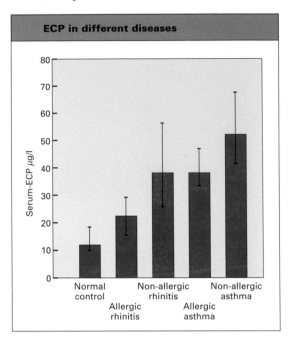

Fig. 4.5 Serum ECP can be used as a measure of the activated eosinophil population. (From Dahl R, Venge P. Role of the eosinophil in bronchial asthma. *Eur J Respir Dis* 1982; **63**(suppl 122): 23–8.)

Chapter 5: The gastro-intestinal tract and food sensitivity

Food allergy is a *controversial subject*, and there is a wide discrepancy between the public perception of food-induced reactions and the medical profession's view of the problem. About 5% of an adult population claim that they react adversely to specific foods, but it is only a minority of these cases which can be confirmed by objective challenge testing.

When people become ill, repeatedly and predictably, when they eat certain foods, they will usually call this 'food allergy'. As adverse reactions to food can be based both on an immunological and on a non-immunological mechanism, the physician should try to distinguish between *food allergy* and *food intolerance* (immunological aetiology unproven or unlikely).

Foods causing adverse reactions

Cow's milk is a prime offender in *infancy*, causing *gastro-intestinal, skin and airway symptoms*. It remains a major cause of allergy into childhood, while allergy to milk is rare in adulthood. The allergenic proteins are *resistant to heating* so cooking milk will seldom reduce its allergenicity. Patients allergic to cow's milk will also react to *goat's milk. IgE antibody* can be demonstrated in most patients with clinical sensitivity to cow's milk protein, but it is possible that *IgG antibody* plays a role in a few cases.

Hen's eggs. Allergy to hen's eggs is important, especially in children. The major allergens are contained in the *egg white.* Most proteins are *resistant to heat* and allergic persons will therefore react to both raw and cooked eggs.

Fish. This contains very *potent allergens* and can, within minutes, cause angioedema, urticaria, gastro-intestinal symptoms, asthma and anaphylactic reactions. The diagnosis is easy as all cases are *IgE-mediated.* About 50% of fish-allergic patients react to all species, while 50% tolerate some species of fish.

Cereals. *Wheat, rye* and *barley* are occasionally involved in allergic reactions in which gastro-intestinal symptoms predominate. Belonging to the same family they exhibit pronounced cross-reactivity. *Wheat flour protein* can cause three types of disease: (1) food allergy; (2) inhalant allergy (baker's asthma); and (3) gluten enteropathy (coeliac disease). A patient with inhalant allergy may not react to ingestion of the allergen and vice versa.

Peanuts. These have long been noted as a *potent allergen* capable of eliciting life-threatening *anaphylactic reactions.* While the allergen is obvious in roasted peanuts and in peanut butter, it can be hidden from the patient as a nutritional supplement added to a series of foods.

Soyabean. Soya products, used *in a growing number of foods* (burgers, pre-cooked meals), can cause allergic and anaphylactic reactions.

Shellfish. Shellfish include two families, crustaceans (shrimps, prawns, crabs, lobsters and crayfish) and molluscs (clams, scallops, oysters, and mussels). Most important are the *crustaceans*. Allergens in this family are usually shared by all or most of the members. Crustaceans are noted for their tendency to cause violent allergic reactions of the *urticaria/angioedema* type and occasional anaphylactic reactions. The reaction is *IgE-mediated* and the diagnosis is usually made by the patient.

Nuts. *Cashew nuts* can cause severe anaphylactic reactions. *Hazel nuts* cause itching in the mouth and throat in birch pollen-allergic patients.

Fruits and vegetables. The symptoms of allergy to fresh fruits and vegetables are usually confined to the *mouth and throat*, probably due to enzymatic digestion in the gastro-intestinal tract. Many of these allergens are *heat-labile* and lose their activity when cooked, frozen or tinned. This '*fruit-and-vegetable syndrome*' or '*oral allergy syndrome*' is frequent in pollen-allergic patients due to cross-reacting allergens, occurring in various combinations (Table 5.1).

Citrus fruits are common causes of skin rashes, especially around the mouth, in infants and children with atopic dermatitis. Usually, this reaction is not IgE-mediated.

Beverages. *Alcoholic drinks* often precipitate symptoms in patients with diseases of the gastro-intestinal tract, skin and airways. They contain a series of *biologically active molecules*, dyes, preservatives (e.g. SO_2) and, occasionally, allergens.

Allergen cross-reactivity	
Pollen	**Fruit/vegetable/nut**
Birch	Hazel nut, apple, peach, cherry,walnut, pear, almond, plum, kiwi, potato peel, brazil nut, cashew nut, tomato, carrot
Grass	Bean, lentil, green peas, mugwort, celery, parsley, chives, banana, melon, parsnip, vermouth
Ragweed	watermelon, honey dew melon, cantaloupe, banana, zucchini squash, cucumbers

Table 5.1 Common sensitivities to fruit and vegetables in pollen-allergic subjects due to cross-reactivity.

Tartrazine. This dye, used as a food additive, has been accused of causing urticaria, angioedema and deterioration of atopic dermatitis, and asthma, but it has been very difficult to confirm this by controlled challenge testing.

Sulphites are widely used as preservatives and to inhibit browning in food. There can be high contents of sulphites in *salad bar lettuce*, *wine* and *citrus juice*, and exposure is most likely to occur *in restaurants*. While most asthmatics with hyper-responsive airways react with bronchoconstriction to large doses of sulphites, a small subgroup of patients reacts with *life-threatening asthma or anaphylaxis* to low doses, the '*salad bar syndrome*'.

Monosodium glutamate. This is the active component of seaweed, and it is widely used as a flavour-enhancer in a variety of manufactured and restaurant food. Intake of a large amount of monosodium glutamate can cause the 'Chinese restaurant syndrome' (headache, a burning sensation along the neck, chest tightness and nausea). Some asthmatic patients react with delayed-onset bronchoconstriction to monosodium glutamate, '*Chinese restaurant asthma*'.

Biologically active agents. Foods often contain biologically active molecules. Large amounts of free *histamine* occur in dark-flesh fish. Certain foods have a *histamine-releasing activity* (strawberries, tomatoes, oranges). Other *vasoactive amines* (tyramine, phenylethylamine), which are found in chocolate, red wine and old cheese, can cause headache and urticaria.

Symptoms and diseases

Symptoms caused by food sensitivity typically involve *more than one organ system*. The *gastro-intestinal tract* is affected in most cases, the *skin* is frequently involved, and the *airways* occasionally affected.

Occurrence and natural history. A positive case history of cow's milk-induced symptoms occur in 6–8% of all infants but studies using controlled challenges have shown milk sensitivity in only 2%. About 10% of *asthmatic children* and 30% of *children with atopic dermatitis* appear to have some adverse reactions to food. The frequency *decreases considerably with age* and food reactions are rare in adults.

Allergy to cow's milk *develops in infancy* while allergy to fruit usually makes its first appearance in adolescence. Sensitivity to some foods *often disappears with age*, especially cow's milk (90% has disappeared at 3 years of age), soyabean (90% at 5 years) and eggs (50% at 5 years), whereas sensitivity to others, such as fish, shellfish, peanuts and nuts, usually persists.

Anaphylaxis. Almost any food may cause anaphylactic reactions but those most commonly responsible are *milk, egg, peanuts and soyabean* in children, and *peanuts, nut, shellfish, fish and sulphites* in adults. An anaphylactic reaction can occur when a patient ingests a known allergen, as a *'hidden additive'* to a dish. In a few cases it will only develop when food consumption is followed by exercise, *exercise-and-food anaphylaxis*. Symptoms can have an explosive *onset within minutes* or can be *delayed for up to 1–2 hours*.

Gastro-intestinal symptoms. *Cow's milk* is by far the most important cause of gastro-intestinal symptoms, which may develop when breast-fed infants are weaned on to cow's milk.

The most striking symptom is *vomiting*, followed by *abdominal cramps*, *diarrhoea*, and screaming ('colic'). Recurrent vomiting and chronic diarrhoea can result in *failure to thrive* and even in malabsorption.

Atopic dermatitis. Although about 30% of children with atopic dermatitis have a *positive skin test* and/or show some adverse reactions to food, this is *not the cause of chronic eczema*, but it can induce *pruritus, skin rash and urticaria*.

Urticaria and angioedema. Food allergy is a frequent cause of *acute urticaria* and angioedema but a very rare cause of chronic disease.

Asthma and rhinitis. *Daily ingestion* of food may result in *chronic airway symptoms* in a few *infants and children*, but food is a very rare cause of chronic asthma in adults. The *occasional ingestion* of an allergenic food, however, can cause a severe *acute attack of asthma*, and a few food-sensitive asthma patients run a risk of dying from food allergy.

Rhinitis almost never occurs as the only manifestation of food allergy or intolerance.

Diagnosis

First, *exclude other diagnoses*, for example, gluten intolerance and lactose intolerance. Second, follow a strict testing plan (Table 5.2).

Indication for testing. Testing for food sensitivity is very *time-consuming and demanding*. When no particular food is incriminated by the patient or parents, the diagnostic work will be difficult and a negative result the rule.

Testing can be relevant in infants with significant gastrointestinal symptoms and if cow's milk sensitivity is suspected, in some children with atopic dermatitis and chronic asthma, and in selected adults with the same diseases in a severe form.

Some adults with *atypical symptoms and a firm belief* in food

A simplified guide for diagnosing food hypersensitivity	
Examination	**Comment**
Case history	The patient's case history should point towards a close relationship between intake of a specific food or additive and initiation of symptoms
Symptoms	The symptomology described by the patient should be of the 'classical' atopic type, i.e. immediate allergic symptoms, most often from two or more organs
Allergy testing	Skin-prick testing or *in vitro* testing for specific IgE (RAST)
Diagnostic diet	Symptoms should disappear or at least be significantly reduced by a restricted, tailor-made diet
Challenge	The original symptomology should reappear during challenge; an initial positive open challenge should be confirmed by double-blind challenge
Therapeutic diet	When the diagnosis is certain

Table 5.2 A simplified guide for the diagnosing of food hypersensitivity according to Carsten Bindslev-Jensen and Hugh A Sampson.

allergy come to the physician in order to have their own opinion confirmed. An attempt to obtain an objective result in these circumstances is doomed to failure and the physician is well advised to *avoid testing these people.*

IgE antibody. In principle, a *skin-prick test* and *RAST* give identical results. The usefulness of testing varies with the particular allergen. For fish allergy, for example, the correlation between a positive test and clinical sensitivity is almost 100%. For other allergens, a positive test can be without clinical relevance, and for that reason the *usefulness of allergy testing is limited* in food sensitivity.

Some allergens in commercial extracts may be inactive so it is recommended that they be supplemented or replaced by *fresh foods.* It is easy to make a prick test through a drop of milk, egg white, or juice from an apple, simply to prick the food and the skin with the same lancet, *the prick–prick test.*

Diagnostic trial diet. The diagnostic work is started with daily symptom recording during a 2-week *run-in period* on a normal and varied diet. If the patient has significant symptoms in this period, it is followed by a 2-week *trial diet period* without the suspected food. If the *symptoms improve significantly*, a challenge test with the suspected food is the next step.

Food challenge. An *open challenge* will be *sufficient in infants*, who are unbiased. *In other patients,* an open challenge can be *a first step* in the investigation. If the challenge is negative, testing can be stopped. Otherwise, it is necessary to continue with blind challenges. It has been convincingly shown that, in older children and adults, 50% of all diagnoses will be incorrect unless they are based on *double-blind, placebo-controlled food challenges,* which is the gold standard in diagnosing food allergy and intolerance. This type of testing, however, is *very time consuming* and *involves a certain risk.* Evaluation of the challenge is based on subjective symptoms and, whenever possible, *objective signs* occurring within 2 hours.

Experience with double-blind challenge has shown that the number of foods causing reactions is largely restricted to a short-list including *milk, egg, peanuts, nuts, soyabean, wheat, fish and shellfish*, which account for more than 90%.

Management

Therapeutic elimination diet. The diagnosis should be as certain as possible, as it is difficult to adhere to an elimination diet. When a diagnosis has been established, the patient is informed about the *elimination diet* by *a professional dietician.*

As a general rule, it is easier to avoid 'hidden' allergens and additives when *meals are prepared at home,* using fresh material, than when *prepacked meals* are bought in a supermarket. Most problematic are *restaurant meals.* In those who have had severe reactions, it is recommended that the patients *prepare their own food* from fresh raw materials and avoid factory food.

It is another general principle that the *strictness of the diet* should be *balanced against the sensitivity* of the patient and the severity of the symptoms. Patients who are highly sensitive and have had serious reactions must painstakingly adhere to the diet.

They can be advised to use an *oral mucosa challenge test* if they are served a meal of uncertain composition. If chewing a small amount of the food and keeping it in the mouth for a few minutes results in oral pruritus, the dish must not be eaten.

In *infants allergic to cow's milk*, weaned from breast-feeding, the safest replacements are hypo-allergenic *milk hydrolysate formulae*, but these are expensive. It is important to reconsider the need for the diet at regular intervals. This is of particular importance in the first years of life, because of the *transient nature of adverse food reactions in children*. In infants and young children it is important to eliminate as few foods, for as short a period of time as possible, due to the risk of malnutrition.

Drug treatment. Patients who have experienced life-threatening attacks need adrenaline for self-administration. Antihistamines are effective on oral allergy symptoms, skin itching and urticaria.

Chapter 6: Atopic dermatitis

Aetiology and pathogenesis
Atopic dermatitis is a *chronic relapsing eczema* in *children* and young adults. The skin shows two cardinal abnormalities, a markedly reduced threshold for *itching*, and excessive *dryness*.

Immunological abnormalities. *T lymphocytes accumulate* in eczematous skin. There is an imbalance between *Th2 cells* and Th1 cells, favouring IgE synthesis (Fig. 6.1). Many patients have increased total serum IgE consisting of *allergen-specific IgE antibody* and of *'no-sense IgE'* (IgE without allergen-specificity). Although many patients develop IgE antibody to common environmental allergens, an antigen–antibody reaction is not a major cause of symptoms, and atopic dermatitis is *not a truly allergic disease*. The cause of the disease is unknown, but several factors can influence the intensity of the eczema (Fig. 6.2).

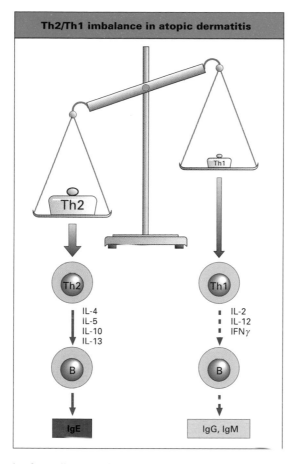

Fig. 6.1 This figure illustrates the immunological imbalance between the two subsets of T helper cells with dominance of Th2 cells having a cytokine profile that favours IgE production in patients with atopic dermatitis.

Skin dryness. Atopic persons with previous or present eczema have an *impaired lipid barrier* in the skin, which leads to an increased evaporation and loss of water, and to dryness and *chapping* of the skin (Fig. 6.3). This is the first step towards irritant eczema, which can be further promoted by intense and prolonged contact with *detergents and irritants.*

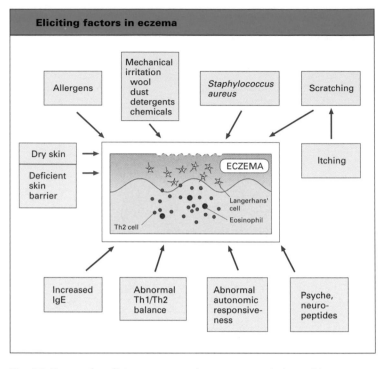

Eliciting factors in eczema

Allergens

Mechanical irritation wool dust detergents chemicals

Staphylococcus aureus

Scratching

Dry skin

Deficient skin barrier

ECZEMA

Langerhans' cell

Eosinophil

Th2 cell

Itching

Increased IgE

Abnormal Th1/Th2 balance

Abnormal autonomic responsiveness

Psyche, neuro-peptides

Fig. 6.2 Factors that elicit symptoms and aggravate atopic dermatitis.

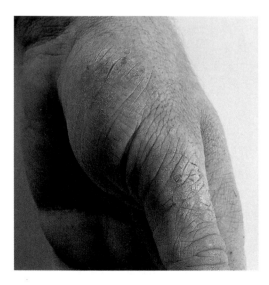

Fig. 6.3 Chapping as a sign of impaired barrier function with increased water loss and skin dryness. The skin is vulnerable, and irritant eczema easily develops.

Clinical presentation

Natural history. The prevalence has *increased considerably* during the last decades, and the cause is unknown. The accumulative prevalence rate (have and have had) is now *10–15%*. The *debut is early*, and 90% have developed the disease before the age of 3 years. The symptoms *usually improve* and *often disappear* (80%) in adolescence, but they relapse in 10–20%. Even though the eczema has disappeared, the skin is still dry and vulnerable, and 25–50% of all children with atopic dermatitis develop irritant hand eczema as adults.

Symptoms. Extreme *itching*, leading to *scratching* and *excoriations*, is the cardinal symptom and it is *not histamine mediated*. All stimuli that increase itching and scratching will worsen the disease and a vicious spiral is started (Fig. 6.4). In the *acute phase*, papules, vesicles and exudation predominate. In the *chronic phase*, the dry skin becomes thickened, lichenified and fissurated.

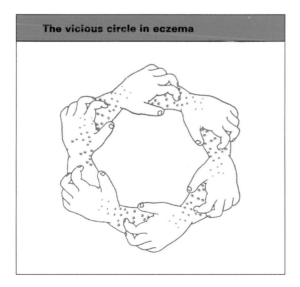

Fig. 6.4 Itching results in scratching which causes more eczema and itching. (By courtesy of Kjell Aas.)

Eliciting factors and complications. There are several factors which can induce exacerbations of eczema (see Fig. 6.2). *Food allergy* may induce an urticarial rash in some patients, but it is not the cause of skin dryness and chronic eczema. Itching and eczema can be induced and aggravated by *skin irritation*, wool, dust, heat, sweating, stress and infection. Both *hot humid weather* and *cold dry weather* are badly tolerated by the patients.

Bacterial skin infections are by far the most frequent complication which must be suspected whenever the eczema starts to ooze (Fig. 6.5). The cause is *Staphylococcus aureus* which, in a lower number, is constantly found on the dry and abnormal skin of these patients. Thus, a positive culture does not necessarily indicate anti-microbial treatment.

Viral skin infections are also frequent complications, and the most important is *herpes simplex virus* (Fig. 6.6). Treatment with an anti-viral compound must be started immediately, even on suspicion of this complication.

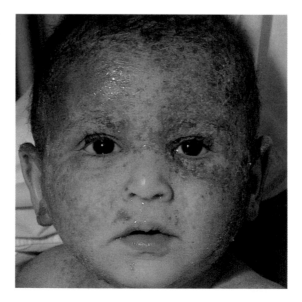

Fig. 6.5 Eczema with bacterial infection. Oozing eczema in atopic dermatitis is often a sign of infection with *Staphylococcus aureus*.

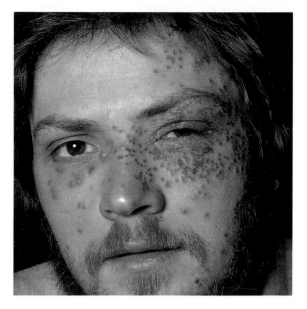

Fig. 6.6 Eczema with herpes simplex infection. This patient with atopic dermatitis developed a herpes simplex infection after contact with a friend having a 'cold sore'.

Infantile stage. Typically, the *scalp and cheeks* are first affected by a pruritic erythema with papules, vesicles, exudation, and, always, *excoriations* (Fig. 6.7).

Childhood stage. This stage characteristically involves the *flexural sides of elbows and knees* (Fig. 6.8), and occasionally the wrists, ankles, neck and head. The extensive scratching often leads to pronounced *lichenification* (Fig. 6.9). *Contact urticaria* to food products, especially oranges and tomatoes, often occurs around the mouth.

Adult stage. A *head-and-neck dermatitis* with red and thickened skin is often added. Allergy to a microfungus, *Pityrosporum orbiculare*, growing in the skin, has been considered as an aetiological factor, but the effect of anti-fungal therapy is only effective in a few patients.

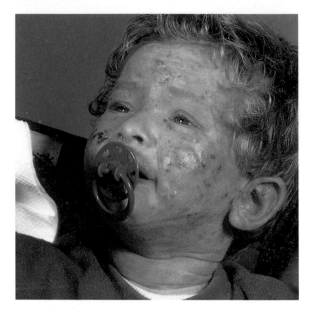

Fig. 6.7 Infant with excoriated eczema in the face.

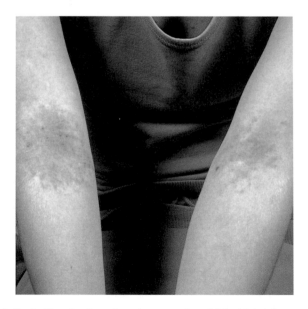

Fig. 6.8 Typical localization of atopic eczema in a child with involvement of flexural sides of elbows and knees.

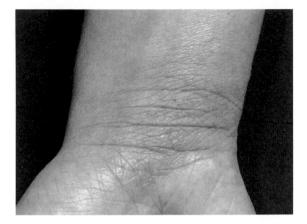

Fig. 6.9 Lichenification of the skin in atopic dermatitis, featuring an increase in visibility of normal skin-markings and thickening of the skin.

Associated diseases. As many as 50–75% of the patients, in particular those with severe eczema, will develop *allergic rhinitis or asthma*. *Atopic keratoconjunctivitis* can be a troublesome complication to eczema in the face (see Chapter 9).

Diagnosis

The diagnosis is based on the *case history* and *physical examination*. In atypical cases it can be supported by measurement of serum IgE and blood eosinophil count. *Allergy testing* is positive in 25–50% of the patients with eczema only, and in 75% of patients with eczema and airway symptoms. Positive reactions to foods may be of little direct significance for the eczema.

Treatment

The therapeutic principles are avoidance of irritants and allergens, and control of *skin dryness, itching, inflammation* and *infection*.

Skin dryness. It is important that the patient uses a *skin moisturiser* on a routine daily basis. Baths with oil are preferable to showers, and the water should be temperate and not hot.

Swimming in sea water and beach life during the summer often have markedly beneficial effects, while bathing in fresh water dehydrates the skin.

Itching. *Cold* is very effective in diminishing itching and the patient should use low temperatures as a remedy: cold showers, cool bedrooms, a walk in the cold evening air, light clothing, etc. *Antihistamines* have an effect on itch in urticaria but not in eczema. However, a *bedtime dose* of a *sedative antihistamine* can be helpful in children who scratch during sleep.

Topical corticosteroids are *the most successful agents* available as they suppress inflammation and itching.

Important for optimal treatment is knowledge about the hierarchy of steroid preparations (groups I–IV based on potency), and of the highly varying skin thickness and sensitivity to steroids in different regions. The palms and eyelids, for example, must be treated differently, because steroid efficacy and side-effects depend upon *epidermal thickness*.

It is an important principle to *start treatment with a relatively potent steroid* and, as soon as disease control has been achieved, to change to a less potent preparation (Table 6.1). In children, in particular, potent steroids should be used for as short a period as possible.

Use of topical steroids in atopic dermatitis
Face and genital area
Group I only (hydrocortisone)
All other areas
Group III (severe eczema) or group II (moderate eczema) —twice daily for 1–2 weeks
Reduce to lower power group —once to twice daily for 1–2 weeks
Group I hydrocortisone on remaining eczema spots —once daily for 1–2 weeks as required

Table 6.1 A guideline for the use of topical steroids for exacerbations of atopic dermatitis.

The major problem is local *side-effects* which will follow regular long-term usage. These side-effects, such as *skin atrophy*, can be severe and disfiguring. In severe cases, however, some side-effects from steroids must be accepted as a price for controlling intolerable itching.

Most parents are reluctant to use steroids on their children, and *underuse* is, therefore, the rule. It is necessary to explain that correct usage not only makes life more tolerable for the child, but it can also reduce scratch-induced damage to the skin.

Tars are the next most useful *anti-inflammatory* agents, but they smell and discolour. Due to irritancy, tar preparations are *not used during acute exacerbation*, and treated skin should not be exposed to direct sunlight.

Skin infection. The best way to keep a low number of *Staphylococcus aureus* on the skin is daily use of *water and a mild soap* even though soap carries a skin defatting and irritating effect. When eczema becomes oozing, as a sign of infection, *anti-microbial bath* therapy (chlorhexidine 0.005%) or fusidic acid applied topically can be recommended. *Systemic antibiotics* are used in eczema with severe oozing.

Diet. There is good evidence that *exclusive breast-feeding* for 4–6 months can postpone the development of some cases of atopic dermatitis, but it is uncertain whether it will be prevented. For the treatment of atopic dermatitis, it is generally agreed that an *elimination diet,* at the most, *plays a minor role.* A patient with eczema on a diet does not become symptom-free, as a patient with hay fever avoiding pollen would. While food allergy and intolerance can cause urticarial rashes in some patients, it is important to emphasize to the parents that it is not the cause of the dry itchy skin or the chronic eczema.

Chapter 7: Urticaria and angioedema

Urticaria (nettle rash, hives) is a disseminated eruption of migrating itching wheals (Fig. 7.1), and *angioedema* consists of similar swellings in the deeper parts of the skin/subcutaneous tissue, and mucous membranes. Urticaria and angioedema often occur together.

Pathogenesis

The lesions of urticaria and angioedema are due to *increased vascular permeability* and *oedema formation. Histamine,* released from *mast cells*, is the key mediator causing increased vascular permeability, vasodilatation and *itching.* In some patients, however, histamine plays a minor or non-existent role (pressure urticaria, cholinergic urticaria, hereditary angioedema).

Histamine release from mast cells can be triggered by IgE-mediated allergy, by other immunological reactions, and by chemical and physical factors. Consequently, there are many causes of urticaria.

Fig. 7.1 Wheals are the typical elements of urticaria.

Causes

An *allergic reaction* accounts for a large percentage of *acute urticaria* but, contrary to common belief, it rarely explains the daily symptoms in *chronic urticaria* (> 1 month).

Idiopathic urticaria. This group, of unknown aetiology, forms at least 75% of all cases of chronic urticaria.

Drugs. *Penicillin* is a frequent cause of an IgE-mediated *Type I reaction*. An IgG-mediated *Type II reaction* can cause an urticarial rash during mis-matched *blood transfusion*. *Type III reactions*, manifested by urticaria, fever and arthritis, can be induced by drugs or by injection of serum, *serum sickness*. Intolerance to *acetylsalicylic acid*, and other NSAIDs, is a frequent cause of urticaria. A variety of other drugs can contribute to an urticarial rash by a direct effect on mast cells (opiates, anaesthetics, muscle relaxants, plasma expanders).

Food. An *IgE-mediated reaction* to food (shrimps, crab, shellfish, nuts, fruits, egg) is a common cause of *acute urticaria* and of an urticarial flare-up in patients with *atopic dermatitis*. Urticaria can also be worsened by foods due to their content of *histamine* (fish with dark flesh) or of *histamine-releasing substances*.

Contact urticaria is due to a direct contact between the causative agent, usually an allergen, and the skin.

Peroral urticaria occurs in food allergy. In a mite-allergic patient with *atopic dermatitis*, contact urticaria can develop when mite allergen is rubbed into the lesioned skin in a mite-infested bed. Contact urticaria of the hands is a common symptom of *latex allergy*.

Toxins. A variety of toxins from *nettles*, *goblets* and *mosquitoes* can directly elicit mast cell degranulation, but immune reactions can also be involved.

Parasitic infections are commonly accompanied by urticaria via an IgE-mediated reaction.

Physical urticaria. Urticaria is characterized by an abnormal responsiveness to physical stimuli. Most frequent is traumatically induced urticaria, *dermographism*, which occurs in all types of urticaria. In some patients, urticaria is selectively induced only by one of the physical stimuli: heat and sweating, cold, pressure, or sunlight.

Cholinergic urticaria develops after *sweating due to heat exposure* or other causes. *The eruption is different* from other types of urticaria and appears as multiple, small papules surrounded by erythema.

Cold urticaria. Attacks will occur within minutes after exposure to cold air or water, bathing or swimming in particular, and this can be associated with anaphylaxis. In a few cases, cold urticaria is secondary to cryoglobulinaemia.

Pressure urticaria. The application of pressure induces *deep, painful lesions*, often localized to palms and feet. The latency time is a few hours, in contrast to the dermographic lesion which develops within a few minutes.

Solar urticaria is a rare disease in which brief exposure to light causes the development of urticaria in the exposed skin area.

Other causes. *Viral infections* may be accompanied by urticarial symptoms but the causal relationship is uncertain and the pathomechanisms are not known. In *malignant disease* (lymphomas) and in *autoimmune diseases*, immune-complex-mediated complement activation can result in *urticarial vasculitis*, which can be diagnosed by a skin biopsy. *Mastocytosis*, with a very high number of mast cells in the skin, is a rare cause of chronic urticaria. Multiple bites from fleas (from cats, dogs or birds) is a cause of *papulous urticaria*, especially in children.

Clinical presentation

The *wheal-and-flare reaction*, visualized by allergy skin-testing or a mosquito bite, is the lesion of urticaria. Wheals are flat, pale-red elevations, surrounded by erythema. They develop within minutes and *disappear within 24 hours* without persistent skin changes. Wheals vary in size from 0.2 to 10 cm and enlarge by peripheral extension to become confluent, with resulting bizarre geographic configurations (Fig. 7.2). Although the lesions *itch*, patients with urticaria *do not excoriate* their skin. Urticaria can develop in any part of the body, often on the trunk, and in particular under *tight-fitting clothing*.

Angioedema (Fig. 7.3) is the *deeper equivalent of urticaria*. It presents as a large swelling and the skin over the swelling appears normal. These elements can persist for more than 24 hours. While urticaria itches, angioedema is felt as tenderness. It frequently develops in the face and mouth.

Urticaria with or without angioedema is common, affecting 10–20% of the population at some time of their lives. The major-

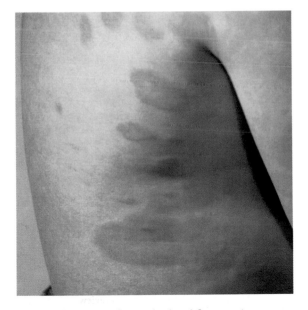

Fig. 7.2 Urticaria showing confluent wheal-and-flare reactions.

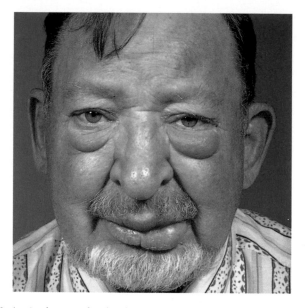

Fig. 7.3 Angioedema is often localized to the face.

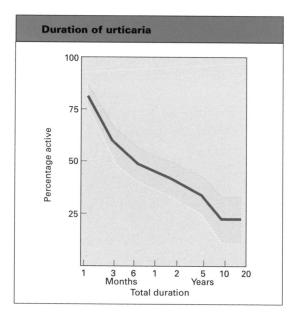

Fig. 7.4 The mean duration of urticaria. (From Champion R, Roberts S, Carpenter R, Roger J. Urticaria and angio-oedema. A review of 544 patients. *Br J Derm*, 1969; **81**: 588–97.)

ity of cases present as isolated *acute urticaria* to foods and drugs. *Chronic urticaria* is most common in middle-aged women. Spontaneous improvement is the rule, even in cases of long duration (Fig. 7.4).

Diagnosis

It is easy to diagnose urticaria in patients with itch and a typical rash. Specific enquiry is directed to ingestion of foods and drugs, *acetylsalicylic acid* in particular.

Laboratory examinations include sedimentation rate, blood eosinophil count, liver and kidney tests, anti-nuclear antibodies, urine analysis, chest X-ray and stool examination for eggs and parasites.

Skin biopsy to exclude vasculitis is indicated in atypical chronic urticaria when the single lesion persists > 24 hours.

Physical challenge tests. Simple challenge tests are available for the diagnosis of physical urticarias. The most common abnormality, *dermographism*, is demonstrated with a blunt instrument or a fingernail (Fig. 7.5). The *ice cube test* can confirm the diagnosis of cold urticaria. An *exercise test* which provokes sweating is a readily available method of producing cholinergic urticaria.

Allergy testing may give information of value in acute but very seldom in chronic urticaria. Patients usually expect to have this examination.

Diet. In selected cases, a diagnostic elimination diet can be justified but, unfortunately, a positive result leading to a helpful therapeutic elimination diet is very rare.

Treatment

Treatment consists of *avoidance* of causative factors when possible, and use of antihistamines. The new *non-sedating H₁ antihistamines* are all highly effective and they have fairly similar

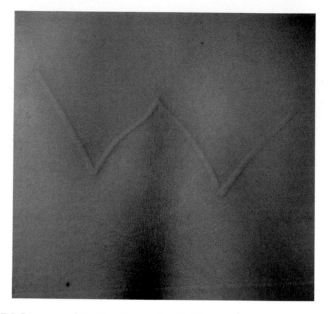

Fig. 7.5 Dermographism ('writing on the skin') is traumatic urticaria seen in patients with chronic urticaria.

effect/side-effect profiles (see Chapter 11). A minority of patients with chronic urticaria, cholinergic urticaria and pressure urticaria in particular, are not sufficiently relieved by antihistamines in ordinary doses. Anxious and frustrated patients with chronic urticaria need confirmation of the benign nature and course of the disease.

Hereditary angioedema

This is a genetically dominant disorder in which the function of a plasma protein, C1 inactivator, is markedly reduced. The angioedema occurs as large swellings in the deeper parts of the skin, and in the mucous membranes.

Mechanisms. The complement cascade can normally be activated by a series of stimuli, and *C1 inactivator* (C1 esterase inhibitor) is the 'break' of this activation. When the 'break' is deficient, complement activation will occur after minimal stimulation. Complement-induced generation of kinins is important for the formation of angioedema, but C1 inactivator is also operational in blood clotting and in the fibrinolytic system.

Clinical presentation. The disease *runs in families* and usually *starts in childhood*. It can involve all parts of the skin, the upper airway and the gastro-intestinal tract.

An attack can occur *spontaneously* or as the result of a minor *trauma*. The swelling, which is tender but not itchy, persists for some days. It is *not associated with urticaria*.

Laryngeal involvement is life-threatening and, in earlier days, was the cause of death in 20% of these patients. A sensation of fullness in the throat, dysphagia and voice change are warning signals. *Dental extraction* and *tonsillectomy/adenoidectomy* can provoke life-threatening oropharyngeal oedema.

Involvement of the intestinal mucosa can cause alarming *abdominal colic*.

Diagnosis. A history of recurrent swellings, starting during childhood, and a positive family history suggest the diagnosis. It can be confirmed by *measurement of C1 inactivator* in plasma (total and functional levels).

Treatment and prevention. The *acute attack* is treated with *adrenaline, intubation* when needed, and in severe cases transfusion of fresh frozen plasma. *Prevention* of the attacks can be attained with *anti-fibrinolytic agents* (tranexamic acid) or *androgenic derivatives* (danazole, stanazole), but the latter are not used in children or pre-menopausal women. Attacks in many patients are sufficiently mild or infrequent not to require long-term treatment but, in every case, *dental work* and *tonsillectomy/adenoidectomy* need pretreatment and observation in hospital.

Chapter 8: Allergic contact eczema

Contact eczema is caused by irritants (irritant eczema), by cell-mediated immune reactions (allergic eczema), or by both.

Immunopathology

Contact eczema resembles immunologically and clinically a true *cell-mediated immune reaction*. Histologically, it is characterized by inflammation with accumulation of activated *Th lymphocytes*, and formation of *microvesicles* in the epidermis.

An *antigen*, as the cause of a Type IV hypersensitivity reaction and inflammation, can be demonstrated in one third of the patients using epicutaneous patch-testing (Fig. 8.1). In the remaining patients, it is probably chronic exposure to *irritants* which induces inflammation by cytokine formation and release from stimulated epidermal cells.

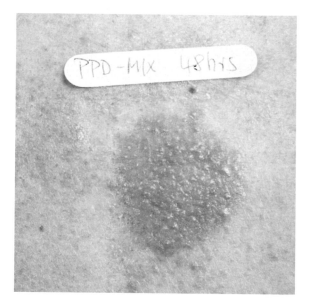

Fig. 8.1 Positive patch-testing. Epicutaneous patch test showing redness and vesicles as a sign of acute contact eczema. This reaction is a sign of cell-mediated immunity towards the antigen in question.

Clinical presentation

Contact eczema is most frequent among women aged between 20 and 40 years. It has probably increased in prevalence, being a concomitant of *atopic dermatitis*, as patients with this disease and dry skin have a considerably increased risk of developing irritant hand eczema.

The course of the disease is often chronic with acute relapses. In the *acute phase* there is severe *itching* and formation of microvesicles in the epidermis (Fig. 8.2). In the *chronic phase*, *scaling and dryness* of the skin are dominant (Fig. 8.3).

Contact eczema usually occurs *in the hands*, where it predominantly develops between the fingers and on the dorsal side of the fingers (areas of thin epidermis and short distance between the environment and the immune system). It can also develop in the face, neck, lower legs and other areas exposed to the antigen and/or irritants.

Occupational contact eczema develops in people with a *high impact of irritants* on their skin. It is advisable to tell children with severe atopic dermatitis that they should avoid the jobs listed in Table 8.1.

The top-10 of dangerous occupations	
Occupation	Prevalence of hand eczema (%)
Cooks and sandwich makers	11
Hairdressers	9
Packing industry	6
Furniture industry	6
Mechanics	5
Bakers	5
Meat industry	3
Fishing industry	3
Laboratory technicians	3
Cleaning assistants	2

Table 8.1 Prevalence of hand eczema in different occupations. (By courtesy of Lars Halkier-Sørensen.)

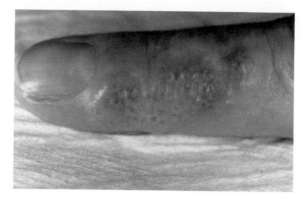

Fig. 8.2 Acute eczema on a finger, resembling the positive patch test.

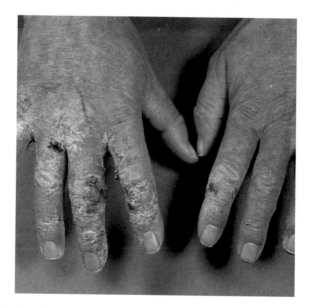

Fig. 8.3 Chronic eczema where scaling is prominent.

Diagnosis

The diagnosis is based on clinical history and examination. *Skin patch-testing* is needed in order to discover possible allergies. Table 8.2 shows a list of the top 10 antigens among a general population. *Nickel* is the most common cause of allergy and ear-piercing is an important risk factor (Fig. 8.4).

The top-10 of contact allergies	
Allergen	Prevalence (%)
Nickel*	6.7
Tiomersal	3.4
Perfume	1.1
Cobalt	1.1
Formaldehyde resin	1.1
Balsam of Peru	1.0
Colophony	0.7
Isothiazolones	0.7
Chromium	0.5
Thiuramix	0.5

Table 8.2 The top-10 list of contact allergies in a general population. * Five times higher in women than in men. (From Nielsen NH, Menné T. Allergic contact sensitization in an adult Danish population. *Ugeskr Læg,* 1994; **156:** 3471–4.)

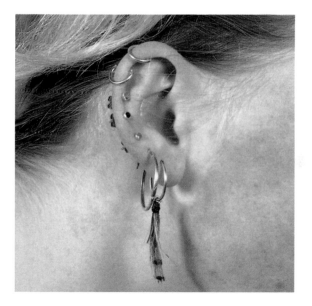

Fig. 8.4 Young lady at risk. Ear-piercing increases the risk of nickel allergy and contact eczema by a factor > 10.

Differential diagnosis: endogenous eczema

Eczema of the hands is not necessarily contact eczema.

An *endogenous form of eczema* is characterized by vesicles in the palms including the palmar side of the fingers. This disorder is called vesicular eczema of the hands, pompholyx (Greek for 'bubble') or dyshidrotic eczema (misnomer).

Relapses will occur within 2–8 weeks, even if the patient avoids all external irritants.

Quite commonly, contact allergies will arise in these patients, and the *eczema becomes a mixture* of endogenous disease, contact allergy and irritant eczema. The course of the disease may be severe and last for many years.

Therapy

Therapy includes *avoidance of antigens and irritants*, and the use of *topical corticosteroids*, which are very efficacious.

Potent steroids should be used once or twice daily until the vesicular eruption is subdued, which may take 1–3 weeks. Intermittent therapy with mild steroids should then be applied. Daily use of emollients will help to prevent skin dryness.

Chapter 9: Eye diseases

Immunology of the eye

It is essential for normal vision that the optical axis passes through *transparent media* only (Fig. 9.1). One can, therefore, understand why the cornea, the anterior chamber, lens and vitreous body all lack lymphatics and blood vessels. It follows that *the eyeball is immunologically deficient*, and the tissues of the eye cannot normally raise an inflammatory response.

The anterior chamber, the lens and the vitreous body are inaccessible to micro-organisms and safe due to their location. The cornea, exposed to the environment, is protected by a structural

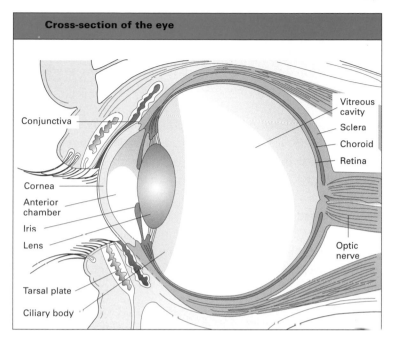

Cross-section of the eye

Conjunctiva

Vitreous cavity

Sclera

Choroid

Retina

Cornea

Anterior chamber

Iris

Lens

Optic nerve

Tarsal plate

Ciliary body

Fig. 9.1 Section of the eye.

defence, the blinking mechanism, tears, and the immune system in the conjunctiva.

As the conjunctiva is fully immunologically equipped, it implies a risk both of allergy and of inflammation. The number of *mast cells* is high in the conjunctiva and the lids, but very low in the lacrimal glands and approaching zero in the eyeball. The distribution of this cell type indicates where allergic diseases are most frequent in the eye.

Allergic conjunctivitis is the eye disease which, with the greatest certainty, can be called an allergic disease. *Vernal kerato-conjunctivitis* is an atopic disease with a significant allergic component. Only these two diseases are regularly seen by the allergist and will be described, but many eye diseases have an immunological background.

Allergic conjunctivitis

This is a common disease, associated in most cases with allergic rhinitis. Eye symptoms are generally more frequent and troublesome in seasonal than in perennial disease, and more significant in allergy to animal protein than in mite allergy.

Pathogenesis. *Histamine*, released from *mast cells* in the *conjunctiva*, is responsible for the principal symptom, itching. Redness is caused by histamine and by rubbing. Tearing can be reflex-initiated from the conjunctiva and from the nasal mucosa.

Symptoms and signs. One of the most troublesome symptoms of hay fever is eye *itching*, which is mainly localized to the medial ocular angle. *Rubbing* gives immediate relief but itching returns and a vicious spiral is started. As a result, the eye becomes *red* and irritated.

Treatment. *Oral antihistamines* can relieve the itching within 30 minutes. *Topical antihistamines* give immediate relief, which lasts 12 hours with levocabastine. The patient should use the drops instead of, and not after, rubbing the eyes. Eyedrops, containing a preservative, should not be used in contact lens wearers.

Prophylactic treatment with *cromoglycate* eye drops every 4 hours can reduce the symptoms, and a simple *eye bath with saline* will also give immediate relief.

It is a sound principle that *only ophthalmologists prescribe steroid eye drops* due to their potential for causing serious side-effects. Short-term systemic steroids can be used when eye and nose symptoms are severe.

Immunotherapy may be considered in severe cases.

Vernal kerato-conjunctivitis

This disease, characterized by *intense itching* and *giant papilla* in the conjunctiva, is chronic with exacerbations during spring and summer, during which keratitis may develop. It is *an atopic but not an allergic disease*, as allergy only accounts for occasional exacerbations and not for the daily chronic symptoms. In this respect, vernal kerato-conjunctivitis corresponds to atopic dermatitis, and the spontaneous course is similar, *commencing in childhood* and, as a rule, *resolving within 5–10 years.*

Symptoms. This rare disease is characterized by persistent and *intense itching* leading to vigorous eye-rubbing, thick, viscous discharge, marked *photophobia* due to keratitis and, in severe cases, impaired vision.

Diagnosis. Examination of the eye reveals *giant papillae* of the upper conjunctiva (Fig. 9.2) and perhaps *keratitis* during exacerbations. The differential diagnosis is contact lens-associated *giant papillary conjunctivitis*, atopic kerato-conjunctivitis and, in some countries, trachoma.

Treatment. Steroid eye drops are necessary but are reserved for acute exacerbations with corneal involvement. Supportive treatment consists of cromoglycate eye drops, antihistamines, antibiotics, surgery, ice compresses and good lid hygiene. Close collaboration with an ophthalmologist is mandatory.

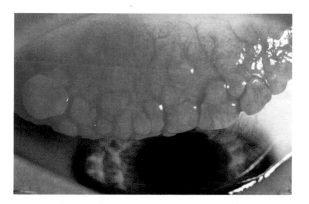

Fig. 9.2 Vernal kerato-conjunctivitis with typical papillary hypertrophy of the upper tarsal conjunctiva. (From Buckley RJ. Conjunctivitis – diagnosis and treatment. In: Holgate ST, Church MK, eds. *Allergy*. London: Gower Medical Publishing, 1993: 20.1–20.8.)

Atopic kerato-conjunctivitis

This is a chronic and very distressing disease of young adults with atopic dermatitis involving the eyelids (Fig. 9.3). It is an adult equivalent to vernal kerato-conjunctivitis, and treatment is similar.

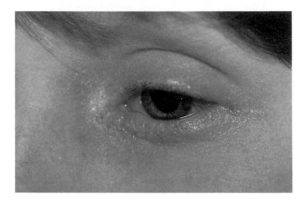

Fig. 9.3 Atopic kerato-conjunctivitis with thickened lid margins and eczematous skin. (From Buckley RJ. Conjunctivitis–diagnosis and treatment. In: Holgate ST, Church MK, eds. *Allergy*. London: Gower Medical Publishing, 1993: 20.1–20.8.)

Chapter 10: Rhinitis: pathogenesis

Structure and function of the nose

The nasal cavities are two 10–12 cm long *slit-like passages* only 2–4 mm wide. The narrowest part of the whole airway is the *internal ostium* (nasal valve), which separates the vestibule from the nasal cavity (Figs 10.1 and 10.2).

The anatomy of the nose, giving close contact between inhaled air and the mucous membrane, is important for its functions: *heating, humidification* and *filtration* of inhaled air. The width of the nasal passages is actively regulated by sympathetic nerves, acting on the venous sinusoids. This permits the nose to adjust itself quickly to changing demands.

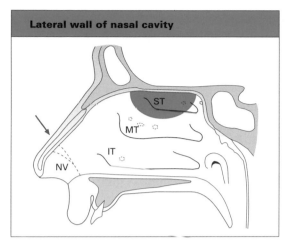

Fig. 10.1 NV is the nasal vestibule and the coloured area the olfactory region. The arrow points to the internal ostium. The openings from the naso-lacrimal duct and paranasal sinuses are under the inferior (IT), middle (MT), and superior turbinates (ST).

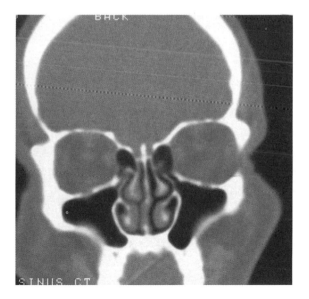

Fig. 10.2 CT-scan imaging of the nose and paranasal sinuses gives an excellent presentation of the anatomy. Note how the mucous membrane in the nose takes shape after the surrounding structures, creating a slit-like air passage.

The sympathetic tone normally changes from one nostril to the other in a 2–4-hour cycle, the *nasal cycle*.

Air conditioning. The mucous membrane supplies water (many glands) and heat (high blood flow) to the inhaled air, and the nose can condition inspired air more effectively than the mouth. Breathing through the nose is preferable when subjects with *hyper-responsive airways* are exposed to environmental challenges, for example allergens, irritants and cold air. During exercise, oral breathing and hyperventilation cause bronchoconstriction due to bronchial heat loss in asthma patients, and this is partially prevented if nasal breathing can be maintained.

Filtration. The efficacy of the nasal filter *depends upon the size* of the inhaled particles. Very few particles larger than 10 µm will penetrate the nose (pollen grains are 20–30 µm), while most particles smaller than 2 µm (mould spores) bypass the nose. The nose also acts as a 'gas mask' by retaining 99% of inhaled *water-soluble gases* (ozone, sulphur dioxide, formaldehyde), and these gases irritate the nasal mucosa.

Pathogenesis of allergic rhinitis

The nose is the site of more allergic symptoms and illnesses than any other organ, due to its effective filtering action for allergens in the inhaled air.

Allergic inflammation in the nose is characterized by accumulation and activation of Th2 lymphocytes, mast cells (of the MC_T type) and eosinophils (Fig. 10.3).

The allergen interacts with mast cell attached IgE, and released *histamine* stimulates sensory nerves and induces reflex-mediated sneezing and hypersecretion. It also, by a direct effect on vascular histamine receptors, causes vasodilatation and oedema formation (Fig. 10.4).

The clinical effect of H_1 antihistamines in allergic rhinitis indicates that histamine accounts for the great majority of sneezing and associated watery hypersecretion, while it seems to play a

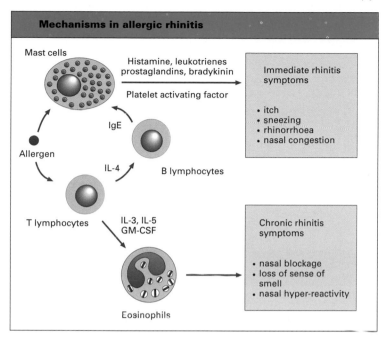

Fig. 10.3 The immunological background of the inflammation in allergic rhinitis. IL-4, produced by Th2 cells (and by mast cells), stimulates B cells to synthesize IgE, and IL-3, IL-5 and GM-CSF selectively recruit eosinophils. (By courtesy of Stephen Durham, National Lung and Heart Institute, London.)

minor role in nasal blockage and no role in hyper-responsiveness, where leukotrienes and eosinophil proteins, respectively, seem to be of importance.

The nervous system. Stimulation of *adrenergic fibres* in sympathetic nerves contracts blood vessels, and *alpha adrenoceptor agonists* (sympathomimetics) are used as nasal decongestants.

Stimulation of *cholinergic fibres* in the parasympathetic nerves causes *hypersecretion*, which is inhibited by atropine and ipratropium.

The sensory nerves in the nose are more exposed to stimulation from cold, dry and polluted *ambient inhaled air* than are the bronchial nerves, and there is a constant reflex activity which stimulates glandular secretion, modulates vascular tone and

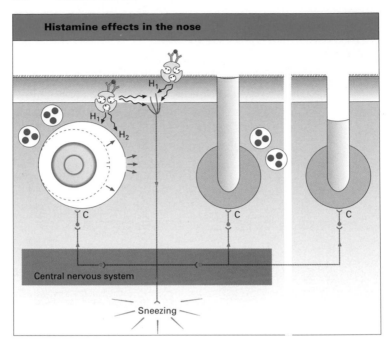

Fig. 10.4 Histamine acts directly on vascular histamine receptors causing vasodilatation (H_1 and H_2 receptors), plasma exudation and oedema formation (H_1 receptors). Histamine stimulates sensory nerves (H_1 receptors) and initiates a parasympathetic reflex via cholinoceptors (C), which results in hypersecretion, also on the contralateral side.

nasal patency. Thus, a certain degree of symptoms can be considered as an expression of *normal nasal physiology*.

Hyper-responsiveness. Both allergic and non-allergic rhinitis are characterized by increased reflex activity and a hyper-reactive mucous membrane. The rhinitis patients, therefore, react with symptoms upon exposure to a series of non-specific everyday stimuli. This seems to be the only abnormality in a subgroup of non-allergic patients (no eosinophilia), while another subgroup has both increased reactivity and inflammation (eosinophilia) (Fig. 10.5).

Rhinitis aetiology, pathogenesis and diagnosis		
Aetiology	Pathogenesis	Disease
Allergy → Inflammation →	Hyper-responsi-veness	Seasonal allergic rhinitis Perennial allergic rhinitis
Idiopathic ? → Inflammation →	Hyper-responsi-veness	Perennial non-allergic rhinitis (eosinophilic)
Idiopathic ? → ? →	Hyper-responsi-veness	Perennial non-allergic rhinitis (non-eosinophilic)

Fig. 10.5 A simplified presentation of the diagnosis of non-infectious rhinitis related to known and unknown aetiology and pathogenesis.

Chapter 11: Rhinitis: drugs

Oral antihistamines

The classical *first generation* H$_1$ receptor antagonists or antihist-amines all have, to a varying degree, a *sedating* effect. *Chlor-pheniramine* and *clemastine* are examples of drugs which cause relatively little sedation and have the highest therapeutic index in this group. They have now largely been replaced by a *second generation* of non-sedating or marginally sedating antihistamines: *terfenadine; astemizole; cetirizine; loratadine; acrivastine and ebastine*. There seem to be only minor differences between the efficacy of these drugs in the recommended doses.

Pharmacology. The drugs are *rapidly absorbed* and are metabo-lized by the hepatic *cytochrome P-450* system (cetirizine is not metabolized but is excreted unchanged in the urine). While the first generation agents readily cross the *blood–brain barrier*, second generation drugs do this with difficulty as they are less lipophilic.

Onset of the antihistamine effect begins within 1 hour of oral administration (astemizole is an exception). It is usually sufficient to give the second generation preparations in *a single daily dose* (acrivastine needs to be given three times daily).

Clinical effect in allergic rhinitis. The antihistamines have a *good effect on itching in the eye and nose*, on *sneezing and watery discharge*, but a *poor effect on nasal blockage*. Generally, they are more effective in *hay fever* than in chronic perennial allergic rhinitis, characterized by nasal blockage.

Side-effects. In most patients, the *first generation* antihistamines will cause *sedation*, impairment of cognitive and psychomotor functions, diminished alertness and slow reaction time. When the *second generation* drugs are given in the manufacturers' recommended dose only a few sensitive patients may experience sedation.

Overdosing with *terfenadine and astemizole* can cause serious *cardiac arrhythmias* (QT prolongation, torsades de pointes, ventricular tachycardia, cardiac arrest and death), which may also result from drug interaction. In order to eliminate the risk of life-threatening cardiac arrhythmias, the patient must adhere to the guidelines in Table 11.1.

Safe use of terfenadine and astemizole
The recommended dose should not be exceeded

Avoid concomitant administration of:
    ketoconazole and itraconazole
    erythromycin and other macrolide antibiotics
    other drugs metabolized by cytochrome P-450 3A4

The drugs are contraindicated in patients with significant hepatic dysfunction
Other antihistamines are preferable in patients with cardiac disease
Discuss the potential risks with the patient

Table 11.1 Measures to eliminate the risk of serious cardiac arrythmias from the use of terfenadine and astemizole.

Increased appetite and *weight gain* can be a problem with a few preparations (cyproheptadine, ketotifen, astemizole).

Topical preparations

More recently, antihistamines for topical use in the eye and nose have been introduced. *Eyedrops* have a very good and instantaneous effect on itching. When *levocabastine* is used twice daily, it is more effective than cromoglycate used four times daily.

Levocabastine and azelastine nasal sprays offer quick relief of itching and sneezing and, when used twice daily, they can prevent the development of these symptoms. Probably, they are most useful in mild hay fever and before known exposure to allergens.

Intranasal corticosteroids

Topical steroids are currently the *most potent medication* available for the treatment of allergic and non-allergic rhinitis. This treatment is now considered first-line therapy in moderate to severe cases of hay fever, perennial allergic rhinitis in adults, and perennial non-allergic rhinitis.

Drugs and drug administration. A part of the drug, applied to the nasal mucosa, will be absorbed into the circulation. However, modern steroid molecules, which are first-pass deactivated in the liver, have a local effect in the nose at a dosage not associated with a significant risk of systemic side-effects (Fig. 11.1).

Beclomethasone dipropionate was introduced in 1974, and *flunisolide, budesonide, triamcinolone acetonide,* and *fluticasone propionate* followed later. There does not seem to be any major differences between these molecules, and the steroid hierarchy, known in dermatology, does not exist in the nose.

Local therapy can be given from a *metered-dose pump spray*, a *powder formulation* and a *freon-propelled aerosol*. A *once daily* medication is sufficient and has good patient compliance.

Seasonal allergic rhinitis. Symptom relief can be achieved within 6–12 hours and be maximal after 2–4 days. A steroid spray

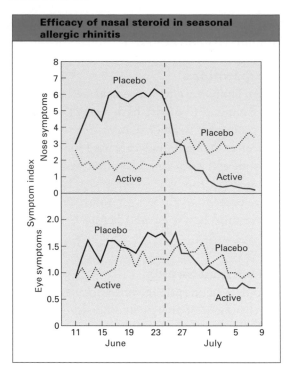

Fig. 11.1 The effect of beclomethasone dipropionate nasal aerosol is marked on nasal hay fever symptoms but absent on eye symptoms, which shows that the mode of action is local and not systemic. (From Mygind N. Local effect of intranasal beclomethasone dipropionate aerosol in hay fever. *Br Med J*, 1973; 4: 363–6.)

controls nasal symptoms in the large majority of patients. There exists no contra-indication to a 2–3-month course of treatment for hay fever in children and in adults. Topical treatment of nasal symptoms necessitates a *prescription for eyedrops* (antihistamine or cromoglycate, *not steroids*).

Perennial rhinitis. Patients with perennial *allergic* rhinitis will get considerable improvement from a steroid spray; the same applies to most patients with perennial *non-allergic* rhinitis and those with nasal *polyposis*.

When nasal blockage is pronounced, a short course of systemic steroids will increase the number of responders. However, a subgroup of patients with perennial non-allergic rhinitis seem to be *non-responders* to any type of steroid treatment. *Nasal eosinophilia* usually predicts a good result.

Side-effects. *Irritation and sneezing* immediately after spraying are frequent but usually diminish with time. *Dryness* in the anterior part of the nose, *blood-stained crusts* and even *epistaxis* can occur but are not progressive and seldom troublesome. Dose reduction, use of an ointment in the nostril and change to an aqueous solution or a powder formulation can be helpful in these cases. Use for 20 years has shown that there is no risk of the development of atrophic rhinitis.

Pros and cons. The *marked efficacy* of intranasal steroids for treating allergic rhinitis is indisputable. It exceeds that of antihistamines and cromoglycate. The major limitation of nasal steroid therapy lies in the relatively *slow onset of action* and the *lack of effect on eye symptoms*.

Safety in children. While intranasal steroids can be used freely in hay fever with a short season, it is the opinion of most paediatricians that their regular use in children with perennial rhinitis should not be a first-line therapy. It is our opinion that nasal steroids can be very useful in moderate to severe cases, in particular when nasal blockage is prominent, and that the treatment is safe, provided the guidelines in Table 11.2 are followed.

Regular use of nasal steroids in children
Daily symptoms of significance for the child
Allergen avoidance carried out
Cromoglycate and antihistamine insufficient
Medication given once daily in the morning
Keep the daily dose as low as possible
Regular checks

Table 11.2 Advice for the use of nasal steroids for perennial allergic rhinitis in children.

Safety during pregnancy. In principle, no medication can be considered as 100% safe during pregnancy, especially during the first trimester. The following rules are advisable: (1) increased restriction in the prescription of any drug; (2) prefer topical to systemic administration; and (3) prefer an old and widely used drug to a recently marketed drug. Use for more than 20 years of topical nasal steroids, given in the recommended dosage, has not been associated with any teratogenic effects.

Systemic corticosteroids

In severe cases, use of systemic steroids is a valuable supplement to other therapies, and a short course can break vicious circles and give prolonged relief. It is a principle that *only short-term therapy* (2 weeks) is used in rhinitis, and when it is not given more than every 3–6 months, the use of systemic steroids can be both safe and useful. In principle, it is not used instead of other treatments but in addition to a basic topical medication.

Preparations. Steroids can be given *orally* (prednisolone, 5–20 mg/day) or as a *depot-injection* (e.g. methylprednisolone 40–80 mg/injection). Oral treatment is confined to 2 weeks, which approximately corresponds to the steroid activity of a single injection. While many general practitioners use depot-injections, most *specialists recommend oral medication*, as the dosage can be adjusted to the changing need for treatment, for example, during a pollen season with a highly varying pollen count.

Seasonal allergic rhinitis. When other treatments are inadequate, the hay fever patient can be supplied with *prednisolone tablets* (5–20 mg daily during troublesome periods).

Perennial rhinitis and nasal polyposis. Systemic steroids, in contrast to topical treatment, reach all parts of the nose and the paranasal sinuses. This treatment can be used to open up a blocked nose before topical therapy and when there is a temporary failure of spray treatment in severe perennial rhinitis or nasal polyposis.

Contra-indications are glaucoma, herpes keratitis, diabetes mellitus, psychic instability, advanced osteoporosis, severe hypertension and tuberculosis. Systemic steroids are not used for rhinitis in children or during pregnancy.

Side-effects from a 2-week treatment are few and mild. Depot-injections can, in rare cases, cause a depression over the injection site. Some authors recommend depot-injections into swollen nasal turbinates and polyps but this must be discouraged as blindness has been reported.

Cromoglycate

Sodium cromoglycate (cromolyn in the USA) can be used prophylactically as a spray in the nose, and as eyedrops. It was originally introduced as a mast cell-stabilizing agent, but its exact mode of action is uncertain. It seems to have a weak anti-inflammatory activity.

Cromoglycate is effective only when used before allergen exposure. Due to its short duration of action, the drug is administered every 4 hours, and that leads to poor patient compliance. Cromoglycate gives a variable degree of symptom amelioration in allergic rhino-conjunctivitis. As it is clearly less effective than topical steroids, the main indication for daily use is *perennial allergic rhinitis in children*. The drug is poorly absorbed and is completely atoxic.

Topical vasoconstrictors

Alpha adrenoceptor agonists contract blood vessels and act as nasal decongestants. They are preferably given topically.

Clinical effect. The potent and long-acting *xylometazoline* and *oxymetazoline*, given from *metered-dose pump sprays*, are easy to use, and to abuse. Patients like the quick onset of action, and the pronounced and prolonged effect (6–8 hours).

Patients not guided by a physician tend to use a vasoconstrictor spray for all types of rhinitis, which is unjustified. It can be used with caution in chronic perennial rhinitis: (1) when the patient starts a basic treatment with topical steroid in order to ensure optimal drug distribution in the nose; (2) when the patient has upper airway infection and sinusitis; and (3) on special occasions when nasal blockage can have detrimental consequences.

Adverse effects. Long-term treatment will result in the development of *rhinitis medicamentosa*, which is characterized by rebound congestion and increased nasal irritability. Regular use of intranasal vasoconstrictors is therefore limited to *7–10 days* and they must be prescribed with caution in patients with a chronic disease. Carefully given information is the best way to prevent rhinitis medicamentosa.

Oral vasoconstrictors

Clinical effect. Oral medication with alpha adrenoceptor agonists has *less effect on nasal patency* than topical treatment but it can be used regularly *without risk of rhinitis medicamentosa.*

Side-effects. It is not elegant pharmacotherapy to constrict every blood vessel in the body in order to treat a stuffy nose, and the dosage needed is at the borderline of that which causes *systemic side-effects* (restlessness, insomnia, tremor, tachycardia, palpitations). There are many *contra-indications* (including coronary disease, hypertension, prostatism, thyrotoxicosis, glaucoma, diabetes mellitus and the use of monoamine inhibitors).

Combined preparations of *alpha agonists and antihistamines* are widely used for allergic rhinitis. These two types of drugs have effects which supplement each other, and their side-effects on the CNS tend to be mutually neutralizing.

Cholinoceptor antagonists

Watery discharge is mediated via cholinoceptors (cholinergic receptors) in the nasal glands. Isolated *watery rhinorrhoea*, not associated with sneezing, rarely responds to antihistamine or steroid therapy. Its quantity can be reduced by topical application of the anti-cholinergic drug, *ipratropium bromide*.

Ipratropium is effective in *perennial non-allergic rhinitis*, but careful selection of patients is necessary, as ipratropium only has effect on watery rhinorrhoea. The spray can also inhibit rhinorrhoea induced by *cold air* ('skier's nose'), *hot spicy food* ('gustatory rhinitis'), and the *common cold*.

The dosage must be adjusted to the severity of symptoms in order to optimize efficacy and minimize side-effects. A significant reduction of attacks of rhinorrhoea can cause a *sensation of nasal dryness* at other times. In that case, a *saline spray* is helpful.

Chapter 12: Seasonal allergic rhinitis

Seasonal allergic rhinitis or *hay fever* is caused by pollen allergy. Pollen grains impinge against the eye and are trapped in the nasal filter, and allergen-containing dust can reach the bronchi. The three important sources of pollen allergens are *trees*, *grass* and *weeds*, which, in the northern hemisphere, have seasons in *spring*, *summer* and early *autumn*, respectively.

Occurrence
Hay fever usually develops in childhood or adolescence, the symptoms remain stationary for 2–3 decades, they will then *improve considerably in middle age* and almost disappear in old age. It is a common disease with a *cumulative prevalence* (have and have had) of *15–20%*, mild cases included.

Symptoms and pollen count
Itching in the nose results in serial *sneezing*. There can be itching in the throat and referred itching in the ears. *Watery rhinorrhoea* necessitates frequent use of a handkerchief. *Congestion* in the nose is usually mild or moderate. *Itching of the eyes* leads to eye

rubbing, and a vicious circle is started, ending with red and smarting eyes.

Some patients, especially those with severe allergy, develop bronchial symptoms at the peak of the pollen season. Patients with *seasonal allergic asthma* often have bronchial hyper-responsiveness all year round. If they are sensitized to perennial allergens, they have an increased risk of developing perennial asthma.

The severity of eye and nose symptoms varies with the daily pollen count, while the correlation is less obvious for asthma. The pollen count is usually *high in sunny, dry weather* and low in cold, rainy periods.

Diagnosis

Diagnosing hay fever is easy. When needed, *skin-prick testing* is usually sufficient to confirm the history, and other examinations are not necessary.

Treatment

Allergen avoidance is not possible outdoors, but excessive exposure can usually be avoided by common sense. The patient's quality of life can be seriously impaired in the pollen season, and as effective and safe therapies are available, the *goal for treatment is a normal life*. Sales figures for hay fever drugs suggest that many patients are under-treated or not treated at all.

Pharmacotherapy. Mild disease with occasional symptoms is treated by *antihistamines* (orally or topically) or by *cromoglycate* prophylactically (Table 12.1).

Moderate to severe disease with daily nasal symptoms is most efficiently treated by a *steroid spray* which is used together with *eyedrops* (antihistamine or cromoglycate). Eyedrops, containing preservatives, can damage contact lenses.

Thus, in hay fever, both nasal steroids and antihistamines can be used as *first-line therapy* in adults and in children. The choice depends upon the frequency and severity of the symptoms and whether they are, predominantly, nasal or conjunctival. A *short*

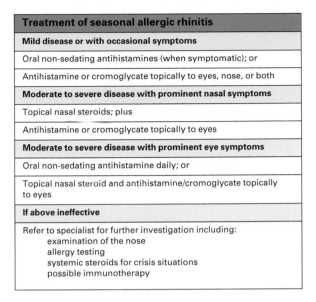

Treatment of seasonal allergic rhinitis
Mild disease or with occasional symptoms
Oral non-sedating antihistamines (when symptomatic); or
Antihistamine or cromoglycate topically to eyes, nose, or both
Moderate to severe disease with prominent nasal symptoms
Topical nasal steroids; plus
Antihistamine or cromoglycate topically to eyes
Moderate to severe disease with prominent eye symptoms
Oral non-sedating antihistamine daily; or
Topical nasal steroid and antihistamine/cromoglycate topically to eyes
If above ineffective
Refer to specialist for further investigation including: examination of the nose allergy testing systemic steroids for crisis situations possible immunotherapy

Table 12.1 Treatment of seasonal allergic rhinitis. (After Lund VJ *et al*. International consensus report on the diagnosis and management of rhinitis. *Allergy*, 1994; **49** (suppl 19): 1–34.)

course of systemic steroids may be added when highly sensitive patients get a symptom break-through at the peak of the pollen season.

Immunotherapy is effective, but opinions vary over when and how often to start this treatment. Most specialists agree that (1) drug treatment should be tried first; and that (2) immunotherapy should be considered when systemic steroids are needed to control the disease.

'Discount therapy'. Economy is a decisive factor in the choice of therapy in many parts of the world. Cheap therapy for hay fever consists of a first generation antihistamine (e.g. chlorpheniramine given once daily in the evening) throughout the entire season with prednisolone tablets added at the peak.

Chapter 13: Perennial rhinitis

Classification and diagnosis

In making the diagnosis, first exclude other diseases and *structural abnormalities* (Table 13.1). Secondly, make a distinction between *infectious* (purulent) and *non-infectious* (non-purulent) disease. Thirdly, separate *allergic* from *non-allergic* patients. The term 'perennial non-allergic rhinitis' is used for a chronic, non-infectious disease of unknown aetiology. Idiopathic rhinitis is an alternative term, preferable to vasomotor rhinitis which incorrectly implies a specific pathogenesis. Fourth, if possible, characterize non-allergic rhinitis as *eosinophilic* or *non-eosinophilic*.

Occurrence

The prevalence rate is about 5%. Allergic rhinitis often starts in childhood while the first appearance of non-allergic rhinitis, as a rule, is in adult life. The course of the disease is capricious and less favourable than that of seasonal allergic rhinitis.

Aetiology and trigger factors

Mite allergy is the most important cause of *chronic* allergic

Differential diagnoses
Mechanical factors
Septal deviation, abnormal ostiomeatal complex, nasal polyps, foreign body, tumours of nose, sinuses and nasopharynx, congenital choanal atresia, meningocele/encephalocele, adenoidal hypertrophy
Infections
Common cold, bacterial infection, sinusitis, leprosy, immunodeficiency, primary ciliary dyskinesia
Miscellaneous
Rhinitis medicamentosa, cocaine abuse, pregnancy, antihypertensive drugs, Wegener's granulomatosis, cystic fibrosis, leak of cerebrospinal fluid

Table 13.1 Other causes of nasal symptoms.

symptoms, and *allergy to animals* (cat and dog) frequently causes *occasional* symptoms. *Pollen* allergy is a common cause of
perennial disease in tropical and subtropical countries. Allergy to
flour is often a cause of isolated rhinitis in bakers, but otherwise
rhinitis due to an *occupational allergen* is usually associated with
asthma. As a general rule, *food allergy* and intolerance *do not
cause isolated rhinitis.* The *aetiology is unknown* in the patients
with negative skin-testing.

All patients with chronic symptoms react to a series of *non-
specific stimuli and irritants*: cold air, dust, fumes, paint, polluted air, printing ink, washing powder, hot spicy food and alcoholic beverages.

Symptoms and signs

Symptoms are largely the same as those of hay fever, but *eye-
itching is less frequent* and *nasal blockage more prominent.*

Some patients mainly complain of sneezing and watery rhinorrhoea, '*sneezers*', while others have nasal blockage and
mucous secretion as dominant symptoms, '*blockers*'. Some
patients, especially elderly gentlemen, have watery rhinorrhoea
as the only symptom, '*runners*'.

Quantitative criteria are necessary to distinguish a minor disorder from a significant disease requiring further examination
and therapy. The average *number of sneezes, number of nose
blowings* and *daily duration of symptoms* are useful measures of
severity.

Examinations

Face and outer nose. The face will often show characteristic signs
in children with perennial allergic rhinitis (Fig. 13.1). If nasal
obstruction is severe, an open-mouthed face is seen, which can
predispose the child to a high-arched palate, overbite and dental
malocclusion (Fig. 13.2). Frequent upward rubbing of the nose
to alleviate itching, '*the allergic salute*', results in the development of a transverse '*nasal crease*' across the lower third of the
nose (Fig. 13.3).

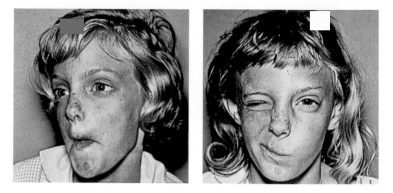

Fig. 13.1 Signs of nasal itching. Mannerisms for relief of itching. (From Marks MB. *Stigmata of Respiratory Tract Allergens*. Kalamazoo: The Upjohn Company, 1972.)

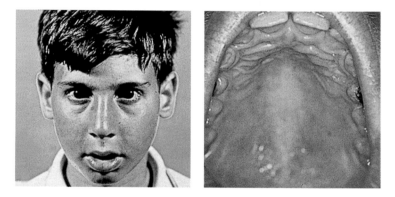

Fig. 13.2 Signs of nasal blockage. An open-mouthed face with a high-arched palate, overbite and malocclusion as a consequence of chronic nasal obstruction. (From Marks MB. *Stigmata of Respiratory Tract Allergens*. Kalamazoo: The Upjohn Company, 1972.)

Rhinoscopy is indicated in all patients with chronic nasal symptoms. It excludes differential diagnosis and can support the rhinitis diagnosis when the mucous membrane is *swollen, wet* and of a *pale-bluish colour*. Rhinologists find that use of a speculum and a mirror provides limited information; they prefer a flexible or a rigid *endoscope*. Nasal patency is estimated by rhinoscopy and, for research, by rhinomanometry, acoustic rhinometry or nasal peak flow.

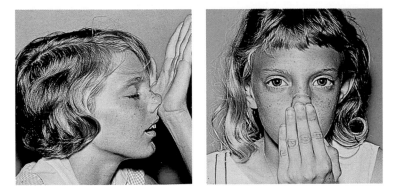

Fig. 13.3 The 'allergic salute' and resulting 'nasal crease'. (From Marks MB. *Stigmata of Respiratory Tract Allergens.* Kalamazoo: The Upjohn Company, 1972.)

Skin testing with a panel of allergens is routine in all patients.

CT-scan imaging provides an excellent tool for the precise diagnosis of anatomical abnormalities, nasal polyps and sinusitis, and for the exclusion of differential diagnoses. It is indicated in selected cases: (1) chronic severe symptoms; (2) for excluding malignancy; and (3) in planning intranasal and sinus surgery.

Nasal cytology is helpful in making a distinction between infectious and non-infectious rhinitis, and between eosinophilic rhinitis and non-eosinophilic rhinitis. A *wiped smear* can be obtained by a tightly wound cotton swab. Better specimens and more reproducible results can be obtained with a *disposable plastic curette* (Rhinoprobe) or a *cytology brush*. When a *rapid staining method* is used the specimen is ready for microscopy within minutes. *More than 10% eosinophils* is suggestive of allergic rhinitis or the non-allergic eosinophilic rhinitis (Fig. 13.4).

Therapy

Allergen avoidance is recommended in animal-allergic patients. In mite allergy, changes in the bedroom may reduce the symptoms (see Table 18.1, page 130). Strict avoidance is more important in children than in adults.

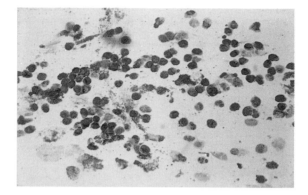

Fig. 13.4 Eosinophilia in a nasal smear as seen in allergic rhinitis and non-allergic eosinophilic rhinitis.

Pharmacotherapy. The drugs used for rhinitis differ in their effect on specific nasal symptoms (Table 13.2).

Antihistamines are predominantly used for occasional symptoms in patients allergic to animals. Patients with daily symptoms will require a *steroid spray*, which is more effective than antihistamines, in particular on nasal blockage. *Short courses of systemic steroids* may be indicated in severe adult cases to open up a blocked nose. Not all patients with perennial non-allergic rhinitis are steroid responders. When watery rhinorrhoea is a dominant symptom *ipratropium* nasal spray is useful.

Drug effect on nasal symptoms				
	Sneezing	Rhinorrhoea	Blockage	Olfaction
Antihistamines	++(+)	++	(+)	−
Oral vasoconstrictors	-	-	++	(+)
Nasal vasoconstrictors	-	-	+++	+
Cromoglycate	++	+	+	−
Intranasal steroids	+++	+++	++	+
Systemic steroids	++(+)	++(+)	+++	+++
Ipratropium	-	++	-	-

Table 13.2 Drug profile in the therapy of nasal symptoms.

In children with perennial allergic rhinitis it is advisable first to try *cromoglycate* together with an antihistamine, and if this is insufficient then to change to a steroid spray.

Other therapies. *Immunotherapy* can be considered in young mite-allergic patients with severe rhinitis and in selected animal-allergic patients.

Surgery of the turbinates can be helpful in non-allergic rhinitis, when medical treatment has failed.

Daily use of an *ointment* in the nostril is beneficial when the skin has become macerated by rhinorrhoea, and *saline* lavage of the nasal cavities can give relief to patients with dry, irritated mucous membranes and viscid secretions ('postnasal drip').

Rhinitis and pregnancy

A persistent *hormonal rhino-sinusitis* can develop in the last trimester in otherwise healthy women; it disappears promptly after delivery.

Chapter 14: Nasal polyposis and sinusitis

Nasal polyps

The polyps, consisting of an oedematously transformed mucous membrane, are pear-shaped with a stalk originating in the upper part of the nose around the openings to the ethmoidal sinuses (Figs 14.1 and 14.2). *Nasal polyposis*, consisting of recurrent multiple polyps, is part of a *hyperplastic rhino-sinusitis* involving the ethmoidal and maxillary sinuses.

Aetiology. This is unknown in most cases. Polyposis is typically associated with *perennial non-allergic eosinophilic rhinitis*, non-allergic asthma and intolerance to acetylsalicylic acid (the ASA

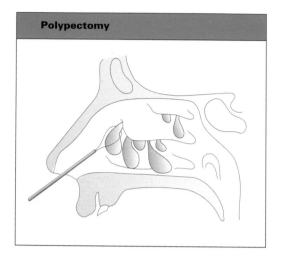

Fig. 14.1 Nasal polyps and a wire snare used for simple polypectomy.

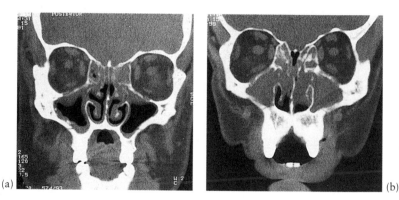

(a)   (b)

Fig. 14.2 Nasal polyposis. CT scan in (a) a patient with early stage polyposis, and (b) a patient with advanced stage of polyposis. (From Holmberg K, Karlsson G. Nasal polyps: surgery or pharmacological intervention? *Eur Respir Rev* 1994; 4: 260–5.)

triad is described in Chapter 2, page 22). Polyps also occur in patients with *cystic fibrosis* and in primary ciliary dyskinesia.

Diagnosis is easily made by rhinoscopy. Nasal polyps are typically *multiple* and *bilateral*. Microscopy is necessary when polyps occur for the first time in order to exclude malignancy, which can masquerade as simple polyps. Microscopy will, in the majority of patients, show a large number of *eosinophils*.

Children with allergic rhinitis do not develop polyposis even though they often have markedly swollen mucous membranes.

A child presenting with nasal polyps needs examination for cystic fibrosis instead of an allergy examination.

Clinical presentation. Nasal polyps, as a rule, develop in a patient who has suffered from *perennial non-allergic (eosinophilic) rhinitis* for some years. *Nasal blockage* gradually develops and can become complete. Impairment or *loss of the sense of smell*, and with that 'taste', is characteristic and very unpleasant. The disease can vary in severity from a single period of nasal blockage to the most severe manifestation of eosinophil inflammation in the upper airways. The reduced ventilation and drainage of the nose and paranasal sinuses predispose to *infectious sinusitis*. Severe cases are usually associated with *asthma*. Questioning about adverse reactions to *acetylsalicylic acid* is obligatory in patients with nasal polyps.

Treatment is a combination of: (1) *long-term local steroid treatment*; (2) *short-term systemic steroid treatment*; and (3) *simple polypectomy*. Combined treatment is often preferable as it prepares the nasal cavity for the intranasal treatment. This basic topical treatment will both improve the rhinitis symptoms and, to some extent, prevent the growth of polyps.

Endonasal *ethmoidectomy* (functional endoscopic sinus surgery or FESS) is indicated in cases resistant to the above treatment schedule.

Sinusitis
Diagnosis. *Allergic children* with chronic perennial rhinitis/asthma have a high incidence of sinus infections, as nasal blockage is a predisposing factor. The hallmarks of sinusitis in children are *purulent nasal discharge*, lasting more than one week, and *night-time cough*. The diagnosis is supported or confirmed by imaging, preferably a CT-scan examination.

Asthma may deteriorate and become more resistant to therapy in children with acute sinusitis. It is not uncommon to mistake acute infectious ethmoiditis for conjunctivitis in a child and this can be serious (Fig. 14.3).

Adults with nasal polyposis have a polypoid, thickened mucosa in the ethmoidal and maxillary sinuses as a parallel manifestation of the basic disease. Their 'radiographic sinusitis' *per se* needs no treatment, unless it is due to accumulation of mucus and pus.

Treatment of acute sinusitis consists of *nasal decongestants, antibiotics* and, when necessary, *sinus puncture.*

In adults with recurrent episodes, surgery is advisable. In this context, the most important area functionally is the *ostio-meatal complex*, localized under the middle turbinate around the openings to the sinuses. It is preferred to use conservative and functional *endoscopic procedures*, which also deal with concomitant ethmoiditis.

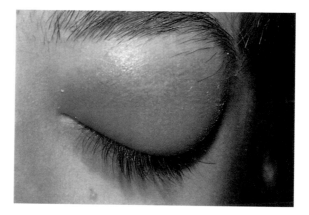

Fig. 14.3 This child does not have conjunctivitis! She was first wrongly treated with eyedrops, but she has acute bacterial ethmoiditis, which in children often is complicated by orbital cellulitis.

Chapter 15: Asthma in adults: pathogenesis

Inflammation

The airway narrowing in asthma is explained by contraction of bronchial smooth-muscle and airway wall thickening due to inflammation (Fig. 15.1). The inflammatory changes in the bronchi are marked in severe asthma but also occur in mild to moderate disease.

Eosinophils are the most characteristic infiltrating cells. Biopsy studies have shown accumulation and activation of eosinophils even in mild asthma.

Epithelial cell damage and shedding. The airway epithelium is damaged or even destroyed by the combined effects of: (1) toxicity from eosinophil-derived proteins (ECP, MBP); (2) squeezing due to bronchial contraction; and (3) excessive stickiness of mucus. *Shedding of epithelial cells* is therefore a constant feature in asthma. As a result the *mucociliary clearance is grossly impaired* for some weeks after a severe asthma attack.

Mucus plugs. In asthma, released biochemical mediators can cause hypersecretion of mucus from goblet cells and from glands, which are also stimulated by a vagal reflex. The increased amount of mucus is not removed because of the *impaired mucociliary transport* and because patients with hyperinflated lungs *cannot cough efficiently.*

Mucus plugs, which occlude the lumen in a large part of the airways, is the most striking feature in autopsy specimens from asthma deaths.

Oedema is another feature of inflammation which contributes to airway narrowing. Histamine and other inflammatory mediators contract endothelial cells in the venules causing gap formation between the cells and plasma exudation with oedema formation. In addition to these physical changes, exuded plasma proteins

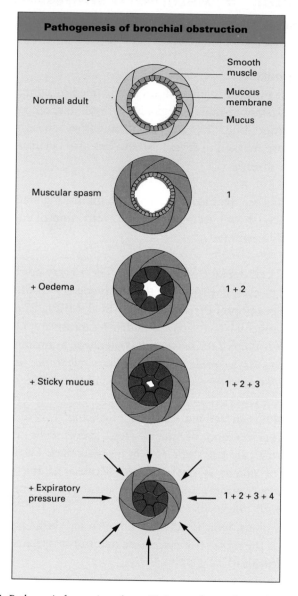

Fig. 15.1 Pathogenic factors in asthma: (1) spasm of smooth muscle; (2) oedema of mucosa; (3) increased amount of mucus; and (4) forced expiration. (From Ass K. *The Biochemical and Immunological Basis of Bronchial Asthma.* Springfield: Charles C Thomas Publisher, 1972: 1–238.)

(complement factors, kallikrein, immunoglobulins) may contribute to asthma pathogenesis.

Other changes. Chronic asthma is associated with: (1) basement
membrane thickening; (2) tissue fibrosis; (3) *thickening of the
bronchial smooth muscles*; and (4) glandular hyperplasia. These
changes in the bronchial tissue may be responsible for the partial
irreversibility of airway obstruction which often occurs when
chronic asthma has persisted for decades.

Bronchial smooth muscle and innervation
There is a spiraling network of smooth muscles around the tracheo-bronchial tree. While its normal function is unknown, it
plays an important role in asthma.

Smooth-muscle receptors. Stimulation of these cell membrane
receptors causes either contraction or relaxation of bronchial
smooth muscles.

Stimulation of the *beta$_2$ adrenoceptor* causes marked muscle
relaxation and bronchodilatation. This receptor is stimulated by
drugs (beta$_2$ adrenergic bronchodilators), by the neurotransmit-
ter, noradrenaline, and by the hormone, adrenaline. The neuro-
transmitter, acetylcholine, released by vagal reflexes, causes
bronchoconstriction by stimulation of *muscarinic cholinoceptors*.

Histamine, stimulating H$_1$ histamine receptors, is a potent
bronchoconstrictor, as are LTC$_4$ and some other mediators.

Sensory nerve endings act as *cough receptors* in the larynx and
trachea, and as *irritant receptors* in the bronchi. They form the
afferent limb of a bronchoconstrictor vagal reflex.

Parasympathetic nerves. There is a dense cholinergic innervation
of tracheo-bronchial *smooth muscles* and glands. Parasympathetic stimulation results in *bronchoconstriction* and glandular
hypersecretion (Fig. 15.2).

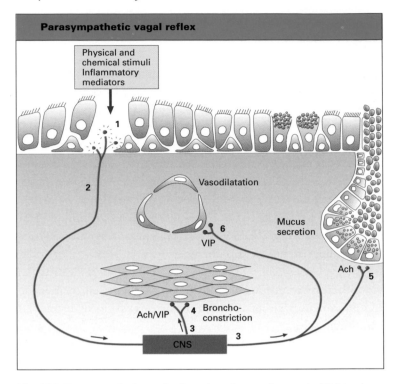

Fig. 15.2 Parasympathetic vagal reflexes in asthma pathogenesis. (1) Stimulation of exposed and sensitized nerve endings by exogenous irritants and inflammatory mediators. (2) Activation of vagal CNS reflex. (3) Stimulation of efferent parasympathetic fibres with release of acetylcholine (Ach) and VIP from nerve terminals. (4) Bronchial smooth muscles are contracted by acetylcholine. (5) Glandular hypersecretion caused by acetylcholine. (6) Slight vasodilatation due to VIP.

Hyperaesthesia. Damage to and *shedding of epithelial cells* in asthmatic airways expose the sensory nerve endings (see Fig. 15.2). They may also be 'sensitized' by certain mediators, such as *bradykinin, prostaglandins* and *cytokines*. In this way, asthma is associated with hyperaesthesia of the airways. Increased neural sensitivity (hyperalgesia) is characteristic of inflammation at other sites in the body.

Smooth-muscle contraction. Mediators, released from mast cells and from other inflammatory cells can cause smooth-muscle contraction by a direct action on the cell receptors. They can also induce bronchospasm by stimulation of tracheo-bronchial afferent nerves and a parasympathetic reflex. It follows that an allergen stimulus can be amplified twice: first, by *mast cell degranulation* and release of mediators; and second, by a *vagal reflex*, which extends the symptoms to sites isolated from the stimulus. Consequently, the interaction between a tiny amount of allergen and IgE can result in a vigorous clinical response.

Receptor activation and smooth-muscle contraction is not only the result of an allergic reaction; it can also be induced by exposure to physical and chemical stimuli.

Pathophysiology

Airway obstruction. Smooth-muscle spasm, oedema, inflammation and mucus plugging cause the prime pathophysiological disturbance in asthma, *airway narrowing* and *increased resistance to airflow*.

Lung hyperinflation. The *use of expiratory muscles* is necessary to maintain adequate airflow through obstructed airways. The increased pressure on the bronchiolar walls closes the distal airways during expiration, and *air is trapped*, leading to lung *hyperinflation*. Bronchial obstruction and air trapping are, in part, compensated for by *prolonged expiration*.

Hyperventilation. During an asthma attack, there is an enhanced drive from the respiratory centre which results in an *increased respiratory frequency* and *hyperventilation*.

Blood gas changes. Hyperventilation results in reduced arterial carbon dioxide tension ($PaCO_2$), *hypocapnia*. In very severe asthma with respiratory failure and hypoventilation, PaO_2 is increased (hypercapnia).

Hypoxaemia is a constant feature of an asthma attack due to a ventilation/perfusion mis-match and PaO_2 reflects closely the severity of the attack.

Chapter 16: Asthma in adults: diagnosis

The case history

Characteristics of asthma. It is difficult to define asthma in exact terms, but the disease has a number of characteristic features (Table 16.1). Clinically it is characterized by *airway narrowing* which is (1) *variable*; (2) *reversible*; and (3) *easily triggered*. These characteristics can be identified by the typical case history, supported by physical examination and, as necessary, by tests, of which the most important are daily peak flow recordings.

The asthma attack is typically described as an episode of *chest tightness*, *musical wheezing* and *dyspnoea*. In patients with mild disease, *cough* can be the only symptom.

Occurrence and natural history. The prevalence rate of asthma is 5–10% (mild cases included). Allergy is an important predisposing factor but only in childhood. Asthma with debut in childhood is usually allergic, while asthma with debut in adulthood is usually non-allergic.

Characteristics of asthma
01 Episodes of wheezy dyspnoea
02 Airway obstruction or narrowing Increased resistance to airflow Reduced ventilatory capacity of obstructive type
03 Rapid and considerable changes in lung function (peak flow variation $\geq 20\%$)
04 Frequent nocturnal episodes and low morning peak flow values
05 Significant reversibility with beta$_2$ agonists ($\geq 20\%$)
06 Significant reversibility with steroids ($\geq 20\%$)
07 Symptom-free periods
08 Frequent occurrence of allergy
09 Eosinophil inflammation
10 Bronchial hyper-responsiveness

Table 16.1 Characteristics of asthma in 10 points.

Asthma *improves in adolescence* in 50% of the cases, but it *often returns* (30%), and allergy is then of less importance. In some cases of severe chronic asthma, *irreversible airway obstruction develops* and the prognosis is dubious due to steadily decreasing lung function.

Two types of triggers. Highly characteristic of asthma is increased bronchial sensitivity (hyper-responsiveness) to a series of stimuli which can trigger an attack. Some triggers merely *provoke an attack* (exercise and irritants are triggers of bronchospasm), while other triggers also *worsen the disease* (allergens and airway infections are triggers of inflammation) (Table 16.2).

Physical examination

In acute asthma, there are *characteristic symptoms and signs* (Fig. 16.1). They have formerly been the only guide to treatment, but now the additional use of objective measurements of lung function are mandatory for arriving at correct management.

A patient with acute asthma prefers to *sit upright with arm support*. *Breathlessness at rest* is a subjective measure, but *speech* is important for evaluation of dyspnoea ('telephone-assessment') (see Fig. 16.1). *Wheeziness* is stethoscopic and often audible at a distance, but it *correlates poorly with airway obstruction*. *Respiratory frequency* and *pulse rate* are better

Triggers of asthma
Triggers that provoke an asthma episode
Cold air, hyperventilation, exercise, laughter, emotional factors, beta blockers, oesophageal reflux
Triggers that also aggravate the disease
Allergens, occupational sensitizers, viral airway infections, tobacco smoke, air pollution, NSAID (a few patients only), severe allergic rhinitis, infectious sinusitis

Table 16.2 Trigger factors which provoke an asthma episode with or without worsening the disease.

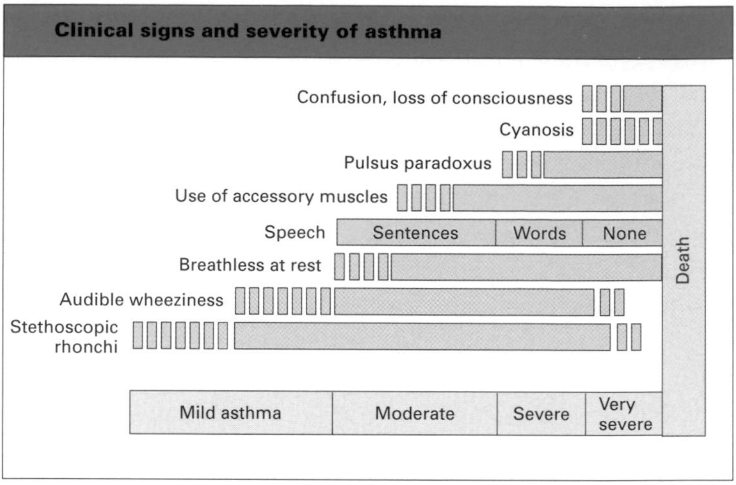

Fig. 16.1 Clinical asthma signs related to the severity of the airway obstruction.

measures of asthma severity. In asthma, in contrast to chronic bronchitis, *cyanosis is a late and unreliable sign* of respiratory failure. Confusion and loss of consciousness herald death.

Laboratory tests

In general, ordinary laboratory tests are not very useful. The *blood eosinophil count* can be helpful in differentiating asthma from chronic bronchitis/emphysema, but a normal count is found in 50% of asthma patients. The eosinophil count is a rough measure of the severity of the disease, and a high eosinophil count indicates steroid requirement. *Serum IgE* is elevated in about 50% of patients with allergic asthma. The *IgE/eosinophil ratio* may be of some help in differentiating between allergic and non-allergic asthma.

Lung function tests

A spirometry curve and measurement of lung volumes in a respiratory laboratory show the principle respiratory changes during an asthma attack (Fig. 16.2).

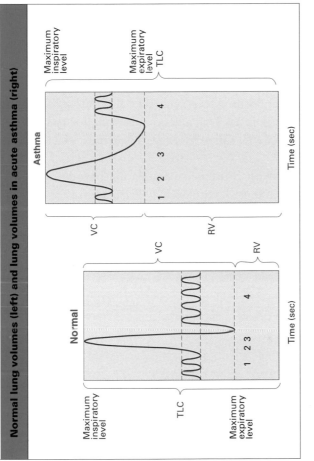

Fig. 16.2 Spirometer curve from left to right: (1) tidal breathing, (2) maximal inspiration, (3) forced maximal expiration, (4) tidal breathing. TLC, total lung capacity; VC, vital capacity; RV, residual volume. Note in asthma: (1) increased residual volume (hyperinflation); (2) reduced vital capacity (dangerous); (3) prolonged expiration (airway narrowing); (4) tidal breathing at a higher lung volume (very unpleasant).

In the clinical setting, repeated measurement of lung function by a simple forced expiratory manoeuvre is the most important observation to be made. It can confirm the diagnosis, detect triggers and assess the severity and response to treatment.

Spirometry measurement. FEV_1 is the single best measure for assessing the severity of airflow obstruction. It can be *measured in the ward* by a dry spirometer. In asthma, FEV_1 is relatively more reduced than the FVC ($FEV_1/FVC < 0.7$), and this is visualized by the 'obstructive look' of the expiration curve (Fig. 16.3).

Peak flow measurement. Measurement of PEF rate by a simple peak flow meter (Fig. 16.4) is a good substitute for spirometry and it is especially well suited for *repeated recordings* and *home monitoring*.

Every patient with chronic asthma should have his/her own peak flow meter and use it regularly. A *PEF diary* is the best way for the physician to obtain quick and precise information about the disease.

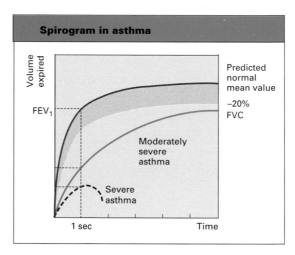

Fig. 16.3 During an asthma attack it is difficult for the patient to 'empty the lungs' (reduced FVC), and especially to do so quickly (relatively more reduced FEV_1). Consequently, $FEV_1/FVC < 0.7$. In severe asthma, only FEV_1 can be measured, as a full forced expiratory manoeuvre induces coughing and bronchospasm.

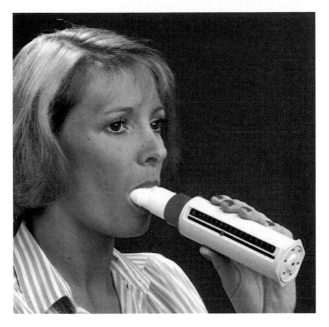

Fig. 16.4 Wright's Mini Peak Flow Meter used for home measurement of lung function (PEF).

Reversibility. A ≥20% *increase in FEV,* 10–30 minutes after the use of an *inhaled beta, bronchodilator* is diagnostic of asthma. Daily PEF recordings, before and after use of a bronchodilator spray, can also be used to confirm the diagnosis.

Exercise test

In most cases, asthma is easily diagnosed by the case history, physical examination, response to a bronchodilator, and daily peak flow recordings. However, a *test for bronchial responsiveness* (exercise test, histamine challenge test) can be a useful supplement in a few cases. These tests require a near-normal lung function (FEV, >70%). The induced bronchospasm can be reversed by an inhaled beta, agonist, which also prevents it completely.

Testing. For clinical routine, the test consists of free running for 6 minutes, sufficiently hard to produce a *pulse rate of 160–180*

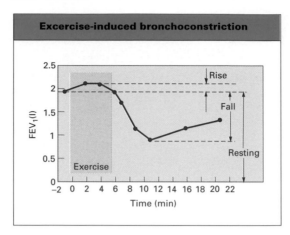

Fig. 16.5 Typical changes in lung function in an asthmatic patient during and after running.

beats/minute. A transient bronchodilatation during the first 2–4 minutes of exercise is, in the asthma patient, followed by a *post-exercise bronchoconstriction* (Fig. 16.5). The test is positive when there is a *fall of ≥20%* in FEV_1 or PEF. This is a test mainly for *children and young people.*

Mechanisms. Exercise-induced bronchoconstriction is due to drying and *cooling of the bronchial mucosa*, and hyperventilation with *cold air* can provoke the same symptoms.

Exercise-induced asthma. Exercise-induced bronchoconstriction occurs in 90% of asthmatics, but clinically, it is mainly a problem in children. While free running is the most potent inducer of bronchoconstriction, *swimming is well tolerated.* Exercise-induced asthma should *not be confused with exertional dyspnoea*, which, in patients with considerable pre-exercise airway obstruction, is provoked by even a modest physical effort.

Histamine challenge test
In adults, a bronchial histamine test (or methacholine test) is preferable for the demonstration of bronchial hyper-responsiveness. It is somewhat *more sensitive* than an exercise test and the

response can be quantified. The histamine test gives an almost complete separation between normal individuals and symptomatic asthmatics, who have a 10–1000-fold increased sensitivity to the provoking agent.

Methods and results. Increasing histamine concentrations are inhaled until FEV_1 *drops 20%*. The Provoking Concentration, causing this fall, is called PC_{20}. A bronchial provocation test should not be carried out when the FEV_1 is $<70\%$ of the predicted normal value. A patient with more than slight bronchoconstriction needs to have his bronchial lability proved the other way round, by bronchodilatation from medication.

Differential diagnosis

Asthma is characterized by episodes of wheezy dyspnoea at rest. Chronic obstructive bronchitis and emphysema or *COPD* is characterized by productive cough and dyspnoea on exertion. In textbooks, and in the typical case, asthma can easily be separated from COPD (Table 16.3).

PEF level and variation. Daily peak flow recordings are important in making a correct diagnosis. They are typically constantly

Is it asthma or COPD?		
	Asthma	**COPD**
Age at start of disease	Child, adolescent	Middle aged, elderly
Smoking	Occasionally	Nearly always
Allergy	Frequent	Rare
Eosinophilia	Frequent	Rare
Dyspnoea at start of disease	Episodes at rest	Exertional dyspnoea
Symptom-free periods	Yes	No
Nocturnal dyspnoea	Yes	No
Normal PEF	Occasionally	Never
PEF variation	$\geq 20\%$	$< 20\%$
Response to beta$_2$ agonist	Good	Moderate and varying
Response to steroid	Good	Poor or none

Table 16.3 Differential diagnosis between asthma and COPD.

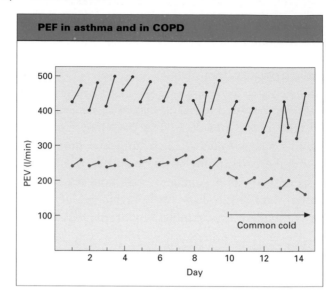

Fig. 16.6 Daily peak flow recordings showing constantly low level in COPD (blue) and high variability (> 20%) in asthma (red). Note the relatively low morning values in asthma. On Day 10 both patients catch a cold.

low in COPD and show more, larger and quicker changes in asthma (Fig. 16.6).

Therapeutic response. In asthma, the airway obstruction is *reversible*, while in COPD it is mainly *irreversible*. In uncomplicated asthma, normal lung function can be obtained, while this is not the case in COPD. The response to a *beta₂ bronchodilator spray* is good in asthma and varying in COPD. The response to *corticosteroid* is good in asthma and poor in COPD.

Mixed diagnosis. In middle-aged smokers with chronic disease it is often difficult to make a clear distinction between asthma and COPD and the diagnosis in these patients is more often 'both…and' than 'either…or'. This is because airway obstruction often is both reversible and irreversible in the two diseases. It is usually said that asthma does not lead to irreversible airway obstruction, but patients with chronic persistent asthma do have an accelerated decline in lung function with age.

Chapter 17: Asthma in adults: drugs

Two therapeutic principles

In principle, there are two types of asthma medication: *anti-inflammatory drugs and bronchodilators*. Bronchodilators were earlier widely used alone as first-line daily therapy and steroid inhalers were looked upon with suspicion. The situation has now changed, and International Consensus Reports recommend anti-inflammatory therapy even in mild asthma and take a cautious attitude to regular use of bronchodilators. Thus, in all but the mildest cases, *basic therapy consists of anti-inflammatory medication*, and *bronchodilators are used when needed*.

The inhaled route is preferred to oral medication due to quicker onset of action, higher efficacy and fewer side-effects.

Drug delivery systems

Inhaled treatment is given by: (1) a metered-dose inhaler (with or without a spacer); (2) a dry powder inhaler; or (3) a wet aerosol nebulizer.

Metered-dose inhalers. In a MDI, the pressurized canister contains the drug suspended in liquid freon or CFC gas. This evaporates when the canister is actuated, releasing the drug as a *micronized powder*. Due to the high velocity, 90% of the particles strike the pharyngeal wall and are swallowed; only 10% enter the bronchi. A *proper inhalation technique* is essential for deposition of these 10% in the lungs and *frequent checks* of patient usage must be undertaken. This type of inhaler contains lubricants which can *irritate sensitive airways*, and frequent use can induce bronchospasm. Due to the well known CFC-induced depletion of the ozone layer in the stratosphere, the *CFC gases will soon be replaced by ozone-friendly gases*.

Spacers. Some patients cannot coordinate actuation of a MDI with inhalation. They can still benefit from inhalation therapy by using a *large volume spacer device* attached to the MDI

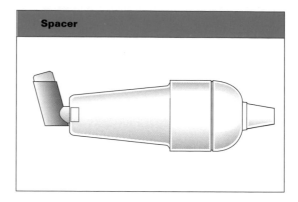

Fig. 17.1 Pear-shaped plastic cone spacer attached to a MDI.

(Fig. 17.1). The spacer allows the patient to *use his bronchodilator spray when asthma is severe*, as he can simply breathe naturally through the spacer. It also reduces drug deposition in the mouth/pharynx and increases it in the lungs.

Dry-powder inhalers. DPIs are as effective as MDIs and they are gaining popularity because they do not contain freon gases or lubricants, and they are easy to use (Figs 17.2 and 17.3). The advantage of DPIs is that the *patient does not need to coordinate* actuation of the inhaler with inhalation. The pattern of deposition depends on inspiratory airflow and varies from one inhaler to the other. While optimal drug distribution is obtained with a slow (1–2 second) inhalation from a MDI, a quick inspiration is recommended with a DPI.

Nebulized wet aerosols. A bronchodilator can be delivered as an aqueous aerosol from an electric nebulizer and this is now the first choice of therapy for *acute severe asthma in hospital*. The use at home is limited by disadvantages: (1) the dose delivered as a wet aerosol is many times larger than that given by a MDI and a DPI; (2) the dosing is imprecise; (3) the electric nebulizer pump and the drug solution are expensive; and (4) the inhalation takes time.

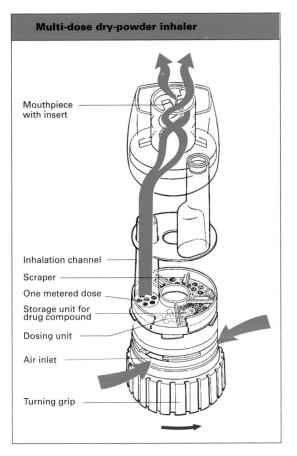

Multi-dose dry-powder inhaler

Mouthpiece with insert

Inhalation channel

Scraper

One metered dose

Storage unit for drug compound

Dosing unit

Air inlet

Turning grip

Fig. 17.2 A powder inhaler is a simple and physiological way to deliver drugs to the bronchi. This device, shown in a sectional diagram (airflow visualized), contains 200 doses of the drug without any additives.

Inhaled corticosteroids

Glucocorticosteroids, corticosteroids, glucocorticoids or simply *steroids* have a broad anti-inflammatory action, which is the main reason for their beneficial effect in asthma. This action is based on a change of cellular protein synthesis, induced by a steroid–receptor complex. Consequently the clinical response to treatment is delayed for some hours.

Inhaled beclomethasone dipropionate, budesonide, fluticas-

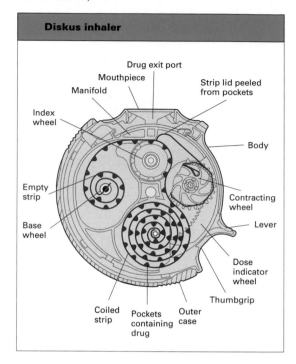

Fig. 17.3 Another example of a multi-dose dry-powder inhaler is the Diskus. It contains 60 doses of drug suspended in lactose, individually foil-blister packed.

one propionate and others *separate anti-asthmatic from unwanted systemic activity*, because they are potent steroids which are quickly metabolized in the liver. Preventive therapy with inhaled steroids is now considered as the most important part of asthma management. It is highly effective and can, in the large majority of patients, completely replace oral steroids.

Delivery system and dosage. Inhaled steroids can be delivered from a *DPI* and from a *MDI with a spacer* attached. Direct use of a MDI is associated with considerable steroid deposition in the mouth and risk of candidiasis.

Treatment is given *bidaily*. It is an advantage that the inhaler can be kept at home and, preferably, be used in the bathroom immediately before tooth-brushing. Gargling and spitting immediately after the inhalation will reduce the amount of steroid swallowed and absorbed.

Low-dose therapy (0.2–1 mg/day of beclomethasone dipropionate or the equivalent) is used for mild–moderate asthma. *High-dose therapy* (1.2–2.0 mg/day) is used in patients with moderate–severe disease, as there exists a dose–response relationship (Fig. 17.4).

Efficacy. Inhaled steroids are the most reliable anti-inflammatory agents for the treatment of asthma and they are *highly and*

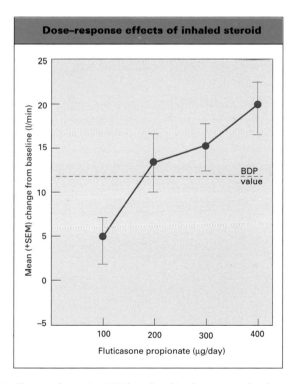

Fig. 17.4 Change of morning PEF from baseline for groups of asthma patients treated with fluticasone propionate compared with the mean value for those treated with beclomethasone dipropionate (BDP) 400 μg/day. (From Dahl R, Lundbäck B, Malo J-L *et al*. A dose-ranging study of fluticasone propionate in adult patients with moderate asthma. *Chest* 1994; **104**: 1352–8.)

predictably effective. Inhalation of 1 mg equals about 40 mg prednisolone orally. It is important to realize the effectiveness, potency and protection offered by a steroid inhaler, as abrupt discontinuation of high-dose inhaled treatment can result in a dramatic loss of asthma control.

The effect on asthma symptoms and lung function starts after days and develops further over months (Fig. 17.5). It may take 3–6 months before full efficacy, for example on exercise-induced asthma, is attained.

Additional use of systemic steroids. Patients on inhaled steroids may need short courses of systemic steroids during acute exacerbations, for example due to an *airway infection. Acute severe asthma* is always treated with systemic steroids, as the penetration and effect of inhaled steroids is uncertain. However, the inhaled treatment should not be discontinued.

Side-effects. *Oral candidiasis* or thrush is a side-effect, especially *from a MDI and from high doses.* It can be prevented by regular

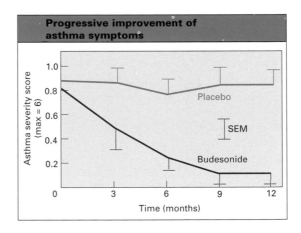

Fig. 17.5 Changes in the asthma severity score. By 12 months, symptoms were reduced to near-zero in the budesonide-treated group. (From Juniper EF, Kline PA, Vanzieleghem MA, *et al.* Effect of long-term treatment with an inhaled corticosteroid (budesonide) on airway hyperresponsiveness and clinical asthma in nonsteroid dependent asthmatics. *Am Rev Respir Dis,* 1990; *142*: 832–6.)

mouth-washing immediately after spraying and the risk is considerably reduced by the use of a DPI or a spacer. Candidiasis is *treated with a local antimycotic*, and it does not necessitate a discontinuation of the anti-inflammatory therapy.

Hoarseness is, like thrush, a side-effect which relates to the dosage. It can be troublesome in some professions (singers, teachers, priests), but it is not progressive.

While low-dose therapy (0.2–1 mg/day) carries no significant risk of *systemic side-effects*, they may occur during high-dose therapy (1.2–2 mg/day), but they are rare and usually mild. When the indication for use of inhaled steroids in a high dose is correct, and when the lowest effective dose is given, then there is no doubt that the benefit for the patient by far outweighs the small risk of systemic side-effects.

Systemic corticosteroids

It is important to realize that while *long-term therapy* with systemic steroids is always associated with a considerable risk of serious side-effects, *short-term therapy* can be given almost without risk.

Steroid reversibility test can be used to show steroid responsiveness and to define the patient's best lung function (for example, prednisolone, 20 mg/day for 2 weeks). Objective *measurement of lung function* (daily PEF) is absolutely necessary to demonstrate the effect.

Short-term therapy. Many asthmatics know when their disease is going to deteriorate (e.g. during a cold), and the prompt use of oral steroids can often abort acute severe asthma. This short-term therapy (2 weeks) can be used liberally.

Long-term therapy is always associated with side-effects and it is used as *the last resort*, and only in addition to high-dose inhaled steroid therapy. While steroids are best used initially in high rather than low dosage, the maintenance dose should be the lowest which can *control the disease*. The dose is *reduced whenever* *possible,* and the potential benefit of oral treatment must always be balanced against the real risk of side-effects. Prednisolone can be given once daily (10–20 mg/day) or as alternate-day therapy (30–60 mg on the second day).

Acute severe asthma. Early use of systemic steroids is an important part of the management of acute severe asthma.

Side-effects. The most frequent side-effects are *Cushingoid appearance* and *weight gain* (Fig. 17.6), and patients must be warned about the increase in appetite. *Sleeplessness* is often a problem when an evening dose is given. The most serious side-

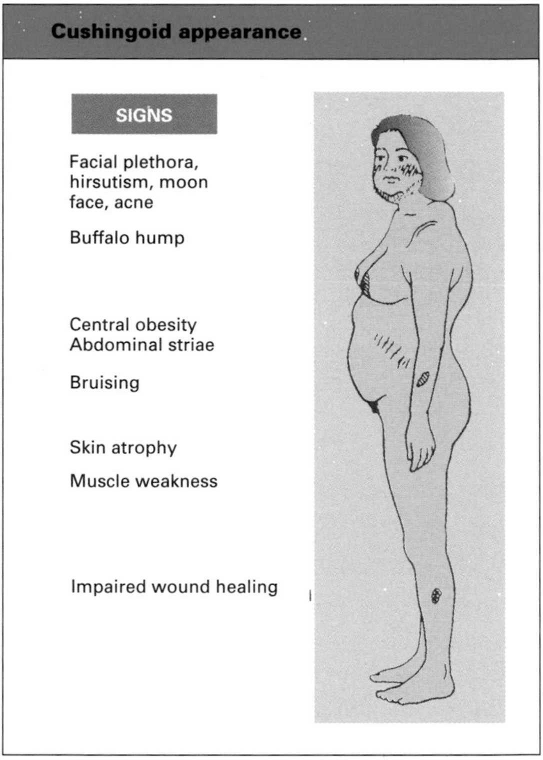

Cushingoid appearance

SIGNS

Facial plethora, hirsutism, moon face, acne

Buffalo hump

Central obesity
Abdominal striae

Bruising

Skin atrophy

Muscle weakness

Impaired wound healing

Fig. 17.6 Signs of glucocorticoid excess. (Idea by Robert P Schleimer, Johns Hopkins University.)

effects are *growth inhibition* in children and *osteoporosis* with painful *compression fractures of the vertebrae* in adults, in particular, in *post-menopausal women.*

Development of *diabetes mellitus, glaucoma, cataract* and *psychotic episodes* are also potential side-effects. Steroids do not cause peptic ulcer or its complications unless they are given with an NSAID. But they can *mask the symptoms of perforation.*

Oral steroid therapy will often, initially, give a feeling of well-being. When therapy, lasting for more than a few weeks, is stopped abruptly the following symptoms occur: malaise, fatigue, mental depression, myalgia and arthralgia. It is important to inform the patient about these *'steroid withdrawal symptoms'.* Suppression of the HPA axis is seldom a problem.

Cromoglycate

When sodium cromoglycate (cromolyn in the USA) was introduced in the 1960s, it was as a mast cell stabilizing agent. Probably, it is now more correct to consider cromoglycate to be a weak *anti-inflammatory agent.* It is inhaled from an MDI, as a powder, or as a nebulized solution.

Allergen-induced asthma. Pretreatment with cromoglycate attenuates the early and the late asthmatic response to *allergen inhalation* and it ameliorates *exercise-induced asthma.* It is sufficient to inhale the drug a few minutes *before* the challenge, but the effect is short-lasting (a few hours).

Clinical use. Cromoglycate is a *prophylactic agent* without effect on actual symptoms. It can be used either occasionally *before allergen exposure and exercise,* or on a regular basis four times daily. It is usually clinically effective in young allergic patients with mild to moderate asthma, but the effect is poor in chronic severe asthma and in non-allergic asthma. Cromoglycate is very safe, but it is clearly less effective than inhaled steroids even in a low dose. As time has shown this treatment to be very safe too, we find it difficult to define a place for cromoglycate in the management of chronic asthma.

Other compounds. *Nedocromil sodium* (nedocromil) seems to be effective also in some non-allergic patients, but the degree of efficacy is similar to that obtained with cromoglycate. Other so-called 'anti-allergic drugs' (ketotifen, tranilast) are widely used in some countries, but the documentation of efficacy is not convincing.

Sympathomimetic bronchodilators

Alpha and beta adrenoceptors. Sympathomimetic drugs can stimulate alpha, beta$_1$ and beta$_2$ adrenergic receptors. While adrenaline stimulates all three receptors, the modern bronchodilators are beta$_2$ selective.

Alpha receptors are predominantly localized to blood vessels. Stimulation results in vasoconstriction, so alpha agonists are used to treat *anaphylactic shock*, *angioedema*, and *nasal obstruction*.

Beta$_1$ adrenoceptors are predominantly localized to *the heart*, and *beta$_2$* adrenoceptors to *bronchial smooth muscles*. As cardiac muscle cells also have some beta$_2$ receptors, tachycardia can be a side-effect of the beta$_2$ bronchodilators.

Beta$_2$ stimulation results in *relaxation of bronchial smooth muscle*, important in asthma, but it also causes *tremor* and a shift of potassium from the extra- to the intracellular compartment (fall in plasma potassium).

Until a decade ago a *cell receptor* was thought of as a 'keyhole' fitting to the specific 'key', the agonist. Molecular biologists have now dramatically changed the situation, as they have identified and cloned the genes encoding for the asthma-relevant beta$_2$ receptor, among others. The characterization of the amino acid sequence of the receptor (Fig. 17.7) has created new and fascinating possibilities for asthma treatment in the future.

Short-acting inhaled beta$_2$ agonists. An inhaled beta$_2$ agonist has a *higher therapeutic index* than medication given by any other route, and inhalation therapy plays a key role in asthma. The risk of serious side-effects is very small, even when therapy is aggressive.

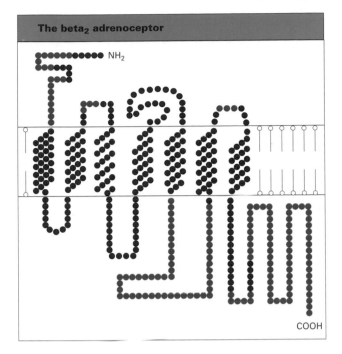

Fig. 17.7 The model for the beta$_2$ adrenoceptor in the cell membrane. Each circle represents a known amino acid. The blue circles are the amino acids which can be replaced without changing the receptor function. (From *Am J Respir Cell Mol Biol*, 1989; 1: 82.)

Inhaled salbutamol or terbutaline produce bronchodilation *within 5 minutes*, which peaks after 30–90 minutes and *lasts for 4–6 hours*. The formerly so popular MDIs are now largely replaced by *DPIs* with no CFC gas and no need for the patient to coordinate activation of inhaler with inhalation.

A short-acting beta$_2$ inhaler is used on an 'as-needed' basis for *episodes of asthma* and for the pretreatment of exercise-induced bronchoconstriction. A large number of inhalations, while not dangerous in themselves, is a warning signal that the control of the disease is deteriorating. Therefore, *when there is a need for regular daily bronchodilator treatment, a steroid inhaler should be prescribed.*

A *spacer* attached to a MDI is useful, *when asthma is severe.* The patient can then inhale repeated puffs of the beta$_2$ bronchodilator without changing his/her breathing pattern. An *aqueous aerosol* from a nebulizer is now the first choice of treatment for *acute severe asthma* in hospital.

Long-acting inhaled beta₂ agonists. These drugs (salmeterol, formoterol) bronchodilate *for more than 12 hours*. They are particularly effective in the *prevention of nocturnal asthma* (Fig. 17.8). Patients still need to have a short-acting beta₂ agonist which can serve as rescue medication for acute attacks, but it is rarely needed due to the high efficacy of the long-acting inhalers. It is emphasized in International Consensus Reports that patients who are on regular bronchodilator treatment also need anti-inflammatory medication (inhaled steroid).

Oral treatment. An oral beta₂ agonist (terbutaline, salbutamol) can be given as a plain tablet or as a liquid formulation, but most

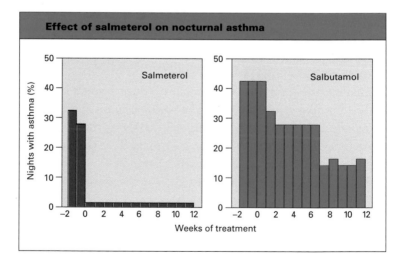

Fig. 17.8 Median percentage of nights with awakenings due to asthma during therapy with salmeterol 25 µg twice daily (left) and salbutamol 200 µg four times daily (right). (From Empye MG, Earnshaw JS, Palmer JBD. A twelve month comparison of salmeterol with salbutamol in asthmatic patients. *Eur Respir J*, 1992; 5: 1062–7.)

often as a *slow-release formulation*. Given twice daily, it produces a moderate bronchodilatation lasting 24 hours. It is usually at the expense of side-effects: *tremor* and *cramps* in the legs.

Oral treatment has less effect on exercise-induced asthma than inhaled beta₂ agonists which definitely have a higher therapeutic ratio. Oral beta₂ agonists can now be replaced by long-acting inhalers in all patients who can master the inhalation technique.

Subcutaneous and intramuscular injection. Injection of salbutamol or terbutaline can relieve bronchospasm within 10–20 minutes. It can be used in acute situations when inhaled therapy is not available.

Intravenous injection and infusion. In *acute severe asthma*, intravenous treatment with terbutaline or salbutamol can be used as an additive to inhalation of nebulized beta₂ agonist. A bolus dose is followed by continuous infusion. *Tremor, tachycardia* and a reduction in *plasma potassium* are side-effects. When intravenous treatment is indicated, a beta₂ agonist is preferable to theophylline.

Cholinoceptor antagonists

A part of the muscular spasm in asthma is caused by a *vagal reflex* via smooth-muscle cholinoceptors, which can be blocked by anti-cholinergic drugs. The inhaled anti-cholinergic agent, *ipratropium bromide,* has a high therapeutic index. It increases lung function significantly for about 4–6 hours but it has a *slow onset of effect*. Mouth dryness seems to be the only significant side-effect.

An inhaled beta₂ agonist is more effective than ipratropium in asthma, but the two types of drug seem to be equally effective in COPD, where ipratropium can be used *together with a beta₂ agonist*. In the initial treatment of *acute severe asthma*, nebulized ipratropium can be a useful addition to a beta₂ agonist. It improves bronchodilatation without contributing to the side-effects of the beta₂ agonist.

Theophylline

This drug has a moderate 24-hour lasting anti-asthma effect, when it is given bidaily as a slow-release preparation. A maximum bronchodilator effect cannot be obtained with this drug owing to the risk of severe side-effects.

Plasma level and metabolism. The plasma level of theophylline is important as it correlates directly with therapeutic and toxic effects. There is a high inter-subject variation in the rate of hepatic metabolism, which furthermore is influenced by a series of factors (Table 17.1).

Side-effects. Mild adverse effects are frequent: *gastric irritation, headache, flushing, restlessness, insomnia* (theophylline minus one methyl group = caffeine), *nausea* and *vomiting*.

High plasma levels (> 20 mg/l or > 110 μmol/l) imply a risk of serious toxic effects: *convulsions* (children) and *cardiac arrhythmias* (adults). As the plasma theophylline level, recommended for high-dose therapy, is 10–20 mg/l (55–110 μmol/l), it follows that the *therapeutic index is very low.*

Factors affecting theophylline metabolism
Reduced metabolism: risk of toxicity
Liver disease
Congestive heart failure
Febrile illnesses
Old age
Liver enzyme inhibition by: cimetidine, erythromycin, oral contraceptives, propranolol, allopurinol and others
Increased metabolism: lack of efficacy
Childhood
Smoking
Liver enzyme induction by: phenytoin, rifampicin, carbamazepine, phenobarbital and others

Table 17.1 Drugs and other factors that influence theophylline metabolism.

Oral theophylline. *High-dose therapy*, aiming at a plasma concentration of 10–20 mg/l (55–110 µmol/l), should only be used by experienced specialists who can *check the plasma level* at frequent intervals. The maintenance *dose is individual* and varies largely.

Low-dose, combined therapy of oral theophylline and beta$_2$ agonist, each in a suboptimal dose, is advantageous because the therapeutic effects, but not the side-effects, are additive. Low-dose theophylline treatment (300 mg twice daily, in a 70 kg adult) can be given without measurement of the plasma level.

Better bronchodilatation with less side-effects can now be obtained with the long-acting beta$_2$ inhalers but oral treatment is still extensively used worldwide.

Intravenous therapy. As theophylline is poorly soluble in water, *aminophylline* is used for intravenous infusion. It is occasionally used in hospital patients with acute very severe asthma. A *loading dose* is followed by an accurately calculated *maintenance dose*. As beta$_2$ agonists, inhaled and intravenously, offer maximum efficacy with few side-effects, the use of theophylline can be questioned, and it has been *discarded* in many departments.

Chapter 18: Asthma in adults: management

Environmental control

Avoidance of allergens and non-specific irritants is *the first measure* to be recommended in allergic airway disease.

Recommendations about allergen avoidance are given to *patients with specific allergies* and to *highly atopic children*, in order to avoid development of new allergies.

House dust mite exposure can be diminished, and the use of mite non-permeable covers in the bed is especially important (Table 18.1). Reducing a high indoor humidity, although difficult to effectuate, is efficient in decreasing the number of mites.

Animals. Avoidance of pet animals is easy – at least in principle. It may take some months after the animal has been removed for the full benefit to be perceived. Indirect exposure from animal protein in other peoples' clothes cannot be avoided.

Air pollution. It may not be possible to avoid *outdoor pollutants*, but avoid exercising in heavily polluted areas. Indoor pollutants such as *wood smoke* and kerosan should be avoided. Passive tobacco smoking provokes symptoms in the majority of asthma patients, and *no smoking* should be allowed in the house.

Daily management

The following programme can be used for the effective management of chronic asthma: (1) definition of the goal for treatment;

Allergen avoidance in bedroom
Let the patient have his/her own bedroom which is used for no other activity
Ban animals and smoking in the room
Accept only a linoleum or wooden floor, which is smooth and easy to clean
Avoid all unnecessary dust-collecting items
Only allow simple furniture and washable drapes
Replace an old box spring mattress with a new one and encase it in an allergen non-permeable cover
Replace old feather pillows with new ones made from a synthetic foam material and encase or wash them regularly
Replace old quilts with new ones and wash regularly (> 55°C or 130°F)
Replace old eiderdowns with new ones and encase them
Clean, vacuum and change bed linen regularly

Table 18.1 House dust mite control measures in bedroom.

(2) daily assessment of asthma severity; and (3) a self-management plan, consisting of a stepwise approach to daily treatment, and an action plan for acute exacerbations.

Treatment goals. Initially the goal for management is discussed with the patient (Table 18.2). The patient's best lung function is defined by repeated recordings, if necessary after short-term prednisolone therapy. The *personal best PEF value* becomes the target for therapy.

Assessment of asthma severity. Asthma severity is currently assessed in order to attain the treatment goal. It is judged by: (1) *symptoms*; (2) *need for beta$_2$ inhaler*; and (3) *PEF*, which is essential. Most patients can be motivated to record PEF measurements daily when they are told that it will enable attainment of the goals of therapy with the least possible medication. Patients with chronic asthma will tend to *under-estimate the severity* of their disease unless they regularly measure PEF.

A stepwise plan for daily therapy allows it to be currently adjusted to the requirement. It is preferable to start on a high step, get full control of the disease, and then step down (Fig. 18.1).

Step 1: short-acting beta$_2$ inhaler prn. The inhaler is used for treatment of occasional attacks and before exercise. Proceed to

Goals for asthma treatment
Normal lung function (> 80%)
Lung function without variability (< 20%)
Minimal symptoms and no nocturnal asthma
No acute severe asthma and risk of death
Near normal life and lifestyle
No side-effects from medication

Table 18.2 Goals for asthma treatment, realistic for patients with mild and moderate disease.

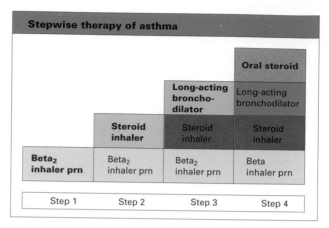

Fig. 18.1 Stepwise therapy of chronic asthma. There are four steps and four drugs.

Step 2 if the patient needs to use the bronchodilator more than three times a week, or if the goal for asthma control is not achieved (Table 18.2).

Step 2: low-dose inhaled steroid. The steroid inhaler is used regularly (≤ 1 mg/day of beclomethasone dipropionate, or the equivalent), and the patients continue to use their beta$_2$ inhaler as needed, but it should not be used on a regular daily basis.

Step 3: high-dose inhaled steroid and regular use of bronchodilator. When initial treatment with inhaled steroids in a low dose does not result in full control of the disease, a high dose (> 1 mg/day) is given. If full control is achieved after 3–6 months, a slow reduction can be attempted, for example, with 3 month intervals. High-dose therapy should not be maintained 'as a routine'.

Patients who need high-dose inhaled steroids for prolonged periods usually have a high degree of bronchial responsiveness. They bronchoconstrict easily in response to exercise, inhalation of irritants and allergens, and at night. These patients will benefit from added use of a *long-acting beta$_2$ inhaler* on a regular basis.

Step 4: regular long-term oral steroid therapy. A few patients with very severe disease cannot be controlled on Step 3 treatment and need oral steroid on a regular basis. Complete control of asthma, as defined in Table 18.2, will not be possible for these patients and the goal of treatment is to achieve a suboptimal control of the disease with as good a quality of life as possible, and as low a dosage of prednisolone as possible. Regular daily use of an oral steroid is *an additive treatment and not a substitute* for other drugs, which should all be given in maximum doses. Repeated attempts to reduce prednisolone dosage and stop the treatment should be made by a specialist.

While regular oral therapy definitely is the final step in maintenance treatment, *short-term oral steroid therapy* may be needed at any level of disease severity.

Action plan for acute exacerbations. It is important that all patients receive a written action plan for acute exacerbations.

Green zone: all clear. *PEF is >80%* of personal best or predicted, and the variability is <20%. There are minimal daily symptoms and no nocturnal symptoms.

Yellow zone: warning. *PEF is 40–80%* and the variability 20–30%. There is frequent coughing, wheezing, chest tightness, decreased activity, and nocturnal asthma. Daily use of a short-acting beta$_2$ inhaler is needed. In this situation, the dosage of inhaled steroid is increased (doubled if possible), and eventually a short burst of oral steroids is given, and tapered off as soon as PEF and symptoms return to Green Zone.

Red zone: medical emergency. *PEF is <40%* and remains there despite repeated use of a beta$_2$ inhaler. The patient needs immediate medical care and, while awaiting the ambulance, should continue to use the inhaler at short intervals, preferably from a spacer.

Acute severe asthma

The earlier used diagnosis, status asthmaticus, is now replaced by the term acute severe asthma, defined by peak flow recordings and clinical characteristics (Table 18.3). Acute severe asthma is usually preceded by a deterioration over some days but severe bronchoconstriction can develop within minutes. As a potentially fatal condition, acute severe asthma must be treated aggressively and observation must be intensive.

Clinical examination. The patient sits upright with arm support. He is wheezing with prolonged expiration, he cannot speak a full sentence, there is tachypnoea and tachycardia.

Lung function tests. *PEF is <40%* of the personal best or predicted in spite of inhaled bronchodilator therapy. However, a patient who can only speak single words may be too distressed to make the expiratory effort.

Blood gases. Measurement of arterial blood gases is *routine* in patients admitted to hospital for acute severe asthma, for grading respiratory function and deciding if and *when to start artificial ventilation.*

Pao_2 *is the best parameter of asthma severity*, and it is reduced according to the severity of the attack (< 8 kPa in severe asthma). The lowest level reached in asthma is about 6 kPa, while patients with COPD can survive even lower levels.

Characteristics of acute severe asthma
Severe dyspnoea at rest
Speech in single words or broken sentences
Relatively prolonged expiration
Stethoscopic wheezes
Tachypnoea ≥25
Tachycardia ≥110
Peak flow <40%
Pao_2 <8 kPa
$Paco_2$ low or normal

Table 18.3 Characteristics of acute severe asthma.

Also $PaCO_2$ *is reduced* in the hyperventilating patient, and an even marginally *raised* $PaCO_2$ *is a very serious sign* in asthma (Fig. 18.2) (not necessarily in COPD).

Due to the short duration of the asthma attack, the $PaCO_2$ changes are not compensated for by the kidneys and arterial bicarbonate remains within normal levels. Increased HCO_3^- and positive base excess suggest a diagnosis of COPD (Table 18.4).

Oxygen must be *given without hesitation*. In asthma, in contrast to COPD, there is no risk of oxygen therapy causing CO_2-retention.

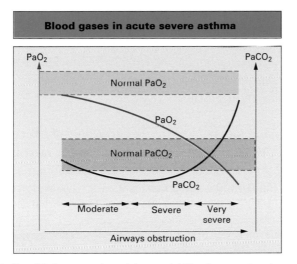

Fig. 18.2 Simplified presentation of the arterial blood gas tensions in acute asthma.

Acid–base disturbances and blood gas values					
	Acid–base disturbance	Pao_2	$Paco_2$	HCO_3^-	pH
Moderate asthma attack	Acute respiratory alkalosis	↓	↓	—	↑
Very severe asthma attack	Acute respiratory acidosis	↓↓	↑	—	↓
Exacerbation of COPD	Compensated respiratory acidosis	↓↓↓	↑↑	↑↑	—

Table 18.4 Acid–base disturbances and blood gas changes in asthma and COPD.

Nebulized bronchodilators. Inhalation of a *beta₂ agonist, repeated* or continuously, in a *high dose* is given immediately by any means, preferably from an *oxygen-driven nebulizer. Ipratropium* can be added initially.

Intravenous beta₂ agonist. If an inhaled beta₂ bronchodilator is given optimally intravenous medication will add little to the effect, but an initial use of two routes of administration can *add to the security* of drug administration. A *bolus dose* of salbutamol or terbutaline is followed by a *maintenance dose* (Table 18.5). Treatment results in tachycardia, tremor and a fall in plasma potassium.

Steroids are obligatory and should be started early, preferably with an *intravenous bolus injection*, which is soon replaced by *oral prednisolone.* High-dose therapy with inhaled steroids is started as early as possible.

Theophylline adds but little to the correct use of a beta₂ agonist, but it can be tried in very severe cases. Dosing must be precise (bolus of aminophylline 6 mg/kg over 15 minutes; maintenance dose 0.6 mg/kg/hour) and contra-indications considered.

Quick checklist in acute severe asthma
Rapid clinical examination
Peak flow measurement
Arterial sample
Oxygen at high flow (at least 4 l/min)
Nebulized salbutamol or terbutaline 5 mg, repeat as necessary, and later every 4 hours, add ipratropium 0.5 mg initially
Intravenous salbutamol or terbutaline 0.25 mg, continue with 10 µg/min (10 mg/l, 60 ml/h)
Intravenous methylprednisolone 40–80 mg, soon replace with oral prednisolone 30–60 mg/day
Re-assess the condition every 2–4 hours (PEF, blood gases, pulse rate, respiratory rate)

Table 18.5 Examination and treatment of acute severe asthma.

Differential diagnosis. Clinically the main problem, for students and professors, is to say whether a patient suffers from *asthma or COPD*. He should benefit from the doubt and *initially receive full asthma treatment.*

Intubation and assisted ventilation is life-saving in a few patients with acute severe asthma. *Call the anaesthetist before* and *not when* intubation is indicated (as described in Table 18.6). Otherwise the decision is based on close clinical observation (*pulse rate, respiratory rate*) and consecutive measurements of *blood gases and PEF.*

It is important for the clinician to know that the interpretation of clinical signs, PEF and blood gas values differs in *asthma and COPD*. An asthma patient with PaO_2 6 kPa and $PaCO_2$ 9 kPa is dying, while a chronic bronchitic patient with similar signs can watch television in the living room.

Treatment during pregnancy

Pregnant asthmatics are concerned about the possible effect of their asthma medication on the fetus. Inform them that ordinary anti-asthma therapy does not imply a risk for the fetus, while severe asthma and hypoxaemia is a real risk for fetus and mother. Acute severe asthma must be avoided at all costs, and if it does occur, the usual intensive regimen is applied. The ordinary anti-asthma treatment is given throughout pregnancy, preferably by the inhaled route, and the pregnant asthmatic should be monitored closely.

Indications for intubation
Cardiac or respiratory arrest
Reduced consciousness
Cyanosis
Patient speechless or can only speak single words due to dyspnoea
Exhausted patient
Hypercapnia (even slightly raised $PaCO_2$)
Severe asthma in spite of aggressive medical treatment

Table 18.6 Call anaesthetist immediately in these cases.

Chapter 19: Asthma death

The old adage that asthmatics never die in the acute attack is not true but the *death rate is low* and most deaths occur in elderly patients.

Insufficient therapy. Half of all asthma deaths occur at home or before admission to hospital. Such *deaths appear sudden and unexpected* to the relatives and even the doctor, but patients have usually had severely compromised lung function for a considerable time. The severity of the airway obstruction has been misjudged and inadequate therapy prescribed or taken.

Sudden, unexpected death. In the rare case, a patient dies within minutes due to *overwhelming bronchoconstriction*. Such patients have often had marked variation of PEF ('brittle asthma').

Death in fulminant status asthmaticus. Even with the best hospital care, acute severe asthma has a mortality rate, but it is low (<1%).

Death in the convalescent period. During the first weeks following acute severe asthma there is a considerably increased risk of death associated with a marked PEF variation.

Overuse of beta$_2$ sprays. Patients with deteriorating asthma use an increasing number of doses from their beta$_2$ inhaler, and this is an important *warning signal*. While asthma death correlates positively with the number of puffs from a beta$_2$ inhaler, it correlates negatively with the use of inhaled steroid. What was needed was not more bronchodilators but steroids to combat the inflammation. Only half of the patients dying from asthma have ever received steroids.

Hypnotics and sedatives. Use of these drugs in acute severe asthma implies a risk of death and is *contra-indicated*.

High-risk factors for asthma death
Brittle asthma with large PEF variation
Low PC_{20} to histamine inhalation
Previous life-threatening attack
Previous attacks induced by food
Prior intubation for asthma
Lack of compliance with therapy
Drug and alcohol abuse

Table 19.1 Characteristics of patients with a high risk of asthma death.

Drug toxicity. *Theophylline* is the only anti-asthma drug which is known to have caused a number of deaths.

Prevention. Asthma mortality and morbidity is still *unacceptably high*. It can be reduced by early use of inhaled steroids, regular measurement of PEF, and identification of high-risk patients (Table 19.1), who should have an open line to a specialist ward.

Chapter 20: Asthma in childhood

Disease and diagnosis

Asthma is one of the most *important chronic diseases of childhood* in the western world. There are a number of anatomical reasons why children, and especially young children, are at *increased risk to airway obstruction*, and more readily than adults develop respiratory failure during acute episodes of asthma.

History taking (Table 20.1). Most of the important information is usually obtained by questioning of *the parents* and that complicates the matter. Parents may be *unaware of important details*

History taking
Family history
General medical history
Atopic history
Environmental history
Specific symptoms
Frequency and severity of symptoms
Description of typical attack
Precipitating factors
Impact of disease on child and family
Physical exercise (play, sport)
School attendance and performance
Psychosocial evaluation
Previous and current therapy

Table 20.1 The history in childhood asthma taken from child and parents.

and they *interpret their observations* and present an 'edited version'. Furthermore, their description of the child's symptoms may be influenced by their *dislike of regular medication*, which they fear has side-effects.

Communicating directly with *the child* is often more useful but not without problems either. Children need *simple, direct and specific questions* and not: 'How is your asthma?' It is important to realize that children with chronic asthma have adjusted their lifestyle to the condition and they consider their *state of chronic invalidism as 'normal'*.

It is often anticipated that asthma is easy to diagnose in children and wheeze is always present, but night-time *cough*, recurrent cough after colds or *unwillingness to participate in sports* may be the only complaint.

Lung function. PEF can be measured by most *children ≥5 years*. However, there is a substantial inter-individual variation in lung function values in children, and PEF can be normal in the presence of quite marked airways obstruction. Therefore, *PEF in per* *cent of personal best after a period of aggressive treatment* is more informative than PEF in per cent of predicted normal.

A *steroid reversibility* trial of 4–6 weeks' treatment with inhaled corticosteroids in a fairly high dose (400–800 µg/day) is very useful in establishing the diagnosis and defining the personal best lung function.

Variability of repeated PEF measurements at home and reversibility to inhaled beta$_2$ agonists are useful as in adult asthma. An *exercise test* is often valuable, while a histamine challenge test is less helpful in children than in adults.

Wheezing illnesses in young children. Wheezing in infants is *extremely common* (about 30%). *Parenteral tobacco smoke* is an important predisposing factor and the most common trigger is a *viral infection*.

There are *two major groups of recurrent wheezers in early life*. In the *transient infant wheezers* (two thirds), wheezing exclusively occurs during airway infections, it is not associated with atopic allergic diseases, and *symptoms disappear* before the age of 3. In one third, it is an *early manifestation of asthma*, and these patients often have: (1) a positive family history of atopic disease; (2) atopic dermatitis; (3) positive skin tests; and (4) symptoms between the episodes of infection-induced wheezing. Without treatment, a *deterioration in lung function* occurs in this group, and they usually *continue to have symptoms* later in life. Furthermore, a large proportion of children with remission in early adolescence will have recurrence of their symptoms when they grow older.

Children with severe chronic asthma show *growth retardation* and *delayed onset of puberty*, but they achieve *normal final height*. By contrast, growth retardation caused by systemic corticosteroids may be permanent.

Drugs and delivery systems

As in adults, pharmacotherapy, given by the inhaled route, is the mainstay in asthma therapy, and oral therapy plays a limited role.

Inhaled therapy. Inhalers and their advantages, disadvantages and limitations will be discussed in some detail with special attention to two important factors: (1) which inhaler is the most simple and *easiest to use optimally?* and (2) which inhaler has the *best therapeutic ratio?* (the therapeutic ratio increases with the proportion of drug deposited in the intrapulmonary airways).

MDIs. Children have *considerable difficulties* with MDIs and thorough tuition is necessary. Most preschool children will not be able to learn effective MDI use. Therefore, *conventional MDIs cannot be recommended for children* when alternative devices are available. A *breath-actuated MDI* abolishes the coordination difficulties and it can be used by children older than 6–7 years.

Actuation during the first part of a deep, *slow inhalation*, followed by a *breath-holding* before exhalation produces the best effect of a MDI. Even when used optimally a MDI results in a *high oropharyngeal deposition* and hence a low therapeutic ratio.

MDI with spacer. Attachment of a spacer to an MDI leads to *reduced oropharyngeal deposition* and increased therapeutic ratio. Spacers are *easy to use,* particularly when they have a valve system. *All school children* can learn to use a spacer and also use it effectively *during acute attacks. Most preschool children* can use a spacer *for prophylactic medication,* but they may not be able to use it efficiently during acute attacks.

Multiple-dose DPIs are easier to use and more convenient than single-dose inhalers. The *inhalation technique is simple.* There is *no need for exhalation before* the inhalation *or breath-holding afterwards.* This is advantageous as *tuition becomes easy.*

The effect of DPIs increases with the inspiratory flow rate, and children should be taught to *inhale rapidly* through these inhalers. Many young children cannot generate a sufficient inspiratory flow rate, and therefore, *DPIs should not by routine be prescribed for children younger than 5 years.* For the same reason, a few older children on powder inhaler therapy may need a spacer inhaler during episodes of severe acute wheeze.

Nebulizers are *expensive and inconvenient* delivery systems. For daily treatment they can usually be replaced by an alternative delivery system. An exception is *children younger than 2–3 years*. A nebulizer is the delivery system of choice for the *in-hospital treatment of acute severe asthma*.

The dose which young children actually inhale to the intrapulmonary airways is lower than that inhaled by the older age groups. *Quiet tidal breathing through a tightly fitting face mask* is normally recommended. Removing the face mask 2–3 cm from the face of the child will reduce the inhaled dose by 50%.

The *therapeutic ratio is low*. Nasal breathing through a face mask will filter off a large proportion of the inhaled particles, which will be absorbed from the nasal mucosa. In this way it may cause systemic effects without adding to the beneficial effect.

Inhaler strategy. Based on the above considerations a simple and yet rational inhaler strategy in children can be outlined (Table 20.2). For *daily use, children ≤5 years of age* can use a *spacer* with a valve system and a face mask, and *children > 5 years of age* can be prescribed a *multi-dose DPI*. For *acute severe asthma*, the patients need a *nebulizer*. It is also used for daily asthma in the few children < 2–3 years old who cannot be taught correct use of a spacer.

Oral theophylline. In general, children metabolize theophylline, as well as other drugs, more rapidly than adults. The *rapid*

Simple inhaler strategy		
Age	Day-to-day use	Acute severe asthma
≤ 5 years	MDI with spacer	Nebulizer
> 5 years	Multi-dose DPI	Nebulizer

Table 20.2 Simple strategy for choice of inhaled therapy for asthma in childhood.

clearance means that children must *take oral drugs at short intervals* or *slow-release preparations* 2–3 times a day. The absorption may be influenced by food.

Children also show considerable inter-individual variation in metabolism and in drug half-life. Consequently, children require *high and individually adjusted doses* of oral drugs to achieve a satisfactory effect, and oral drugs are often used in suboptimal and ineffective doses in children.

Oral beta$_2$ agonists. The bioavailability of slow-release beta$_2$ agonists is lower than that of plain tablets and syrup (30% dose increase). *Food* also reduces the bioavailability (30% dose increase). Optimal dosing with an oral beta$_2$ agonist should be *individualized* based on a dose titration with monitoring of the therapeutic response and the occurrence of side-effects.

Daily management

Treatment objectives. These are: *freedom from symptoms*, a *normal lung function*, prevention of lung damage and a minimum risk of death. The child should be able to live an unrestricted life without avoidance of physical exercise. Although these objectives are achievable in the majority of children they are not fulfilled in many patients. There are a number of reasons for this, including a negative attitude to active pharmacotherapy.

Environmental control. Removal of important *allergens* and irritants such as *cigarette smoking* is even more important in children than in adults.

Immunotherapy may be considered in children ≥ 5 who cannot avoid an allergen of major importance for the disease (see Chapter 21).

Pharmacotherapy strategy. The correct way to treat a child requiring daily medication is still a matter of debate. In principle there are two strategies, the conservative '*step-up strategy*' and the more aggressive '*step-down strategy*'.

The step-up strategy. Treatment is gradually built up using inhaled beta$_2$ agonists, cromoglycate, oral theophylline and oral beta$_2$ agonists. Finally, if added *multi-drug therapy* is inadequate, inhaled steroid is given as the last resort. As only a minority of the children will receive steroids it implies that the child's personal best lung function is not regularly established. Therefore, this strategy implies a substantial *risk of ending up at a suboptimal treatment level*.

The step-down strategy. In this strategy, *inhaled steroids are used early* to establish optimal control and *define the child's best lung function*. A 6–8-week treatment period with high-dose inhaled steroid (800–1000 µg/day) is given, and the treatment is then stepped down every 6–8 weeks to the lowest dose needed to maintain optimal control. With this approach, the majority of children end up on continuous treatment with inhaled steroids. In addition to improvement in quality of life and a reduced morbidity, the step-down strategy also reduces the numbers of acute admissions, increases lung function, and *reduces the risk of undertreatment*.

Beneficial effects of inhaled steroids. In a low dose (≤ 400 µg/day) inhaled steroid is at least as effective as other therapies, and in a high dose (> 400 µg/day) it is definitely more effective. *Patient compliance is good*, due to the bidaily dosing, and the avoidance of multi-drug therapy. More importantly, recent studies have indicated that early treatment with inhaled steroid may *prevent the development of irreversible airway obstruction*.

Potential side-effects of inhaled steroids. *Low-dose therapy*, used for 20 years, seems to be as safe as other treatments. Since our experience with *high-dose therapy* is limited it should be reserved for patients who are not controlled on lower doses in combination with oral bronchodilators or inhaled long-acting beta$_2$ agonists.

Exercise-induced asthma. Participation in sport and play is important for normal growth and psychosocial development of the child. Therefore, exercise-induced asthma is a *bigger problem in children* than in adults. Children with asthma should be *encouraged to participate in all physical activities* and play.

Prophylactic medication with *inhaled beta₂ agonists* and/or *cromoglycate* just prior to exercise is the most widely recommended treatment. However, many children do not know beforehand when they are going to be physically active.

Continuous treatment with *inhaled steroids* and/or *long-acting beta₂ agonists* is helpful, as it does not require premedication immediately prior to the exercise.

Special problems in young children. As there are few controlled studies in young children < 3 years old, the best treatment strategy in this age group is not known. *Oral beta₂ agonists* are widely used but their effectiveness is often disappointing. In contrast, controlled studies with spacers have convincingly shown that *inhaled beta₂ agonists* produce significant bronchodilatation in most children in this age group.

Ketotifen is widely used in young children in many parts of the world, but most controlled studies have failed to justify such use. As for most other drugs, the clinical documentation for *cromoglycate* in young children is more sparse and the results varying.

In contrast to other therapies *inhaled steroids* have been found very effective in young children when administered from a spacer (Fig. 20.1). At present the safety of long-term treatment still remains to be settled in these age groups and, until that has been done, it should be reserved for the more severe cases.

Acute asthma

An acute severe attack of asthma is a *potentially life-threatening* event, which should always be treated effectively without delay.

History and objective findings. The typical symptoms and signs (wheeziness, patient distress, increased respiratory and pulse rates) correlate weakly with lung function and oxygen satura-

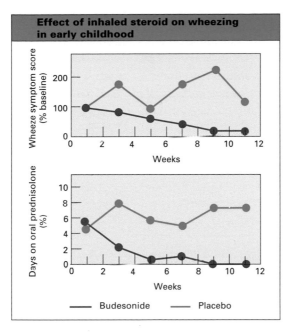

Fig. 20.1 Effect of inhaled budesonide (400 µg twice daily from a spacer) compared with placebo in young children (11–36 months) with recurrent wheezing. *Upper part:* wheeze symptom score. *Lower part:* days on oral prednisolone. (From Bisgaard H, Munck SL, Nielsen JP, Petersen W, Ohlsson SV. Inhaled budesonide for treatment of recurrent wheezing in early childhood. *Lancet,* 1990; **336**: 649–51.)

tion. A quiet chest on auscultation, inability to talk, cyanosis, paradoxical thoraco-abdominal movement and confusion strongly suggest very severe asthma. The asthma *severity is often underestimated* by patient, parents and physician, if objective measurements are not used (Table 20.3).

Blood gases. Measurement of blood gases is a reliable way to assess asthma severity in children. $PaCO_2$ can be reliably measured in capillary blood and is very useful particularly in young children. $PaCO_2$ is low due to hyperventilation during an asthma episode, and a *normal or elevated $PaCO_2$ value should be considered a sign of danger.* An *oxygen saturation* <92% is predictive

Assessment of asthma severity in children			
	Mild	**Moderate**	**Severe**
Treatment place	Home	Home/outpatient	Hospital
Wheeze	Only end-expiratory	Loud	Loud or absent

Breathlessness
  Infant
  Older child
	
	Crying
	Playing
		
		Difficult feeding
		Walking
			
			Stops feeding
			Talks in single words

Accessory muscles, retractions	Usually not	Moderate	Marked

Respiratory rate
  < 3 months
  3–12 months
  1–6 years
  > 6 years
	
	< 60
	< 50
	< 40
	< 30
		
		60–70
		50–60
		40–50
		30–40
			
			> 70
			> 60
			> 50
			> 40

Pulse rate
  < 1 year
  1–2 year
  > 2 years
	
	< 150
	< 120
	< 110
		
		150–170
		120–140
		110–130
			
			> 170
			> 140
			> 130

Pretreatment PEF (%)	> 70	50–70	< 50
$Paco_2$ (kPa)	< 4.9	< 5.6	> 5.6
Sao_2 (on air) (%)	> 94	92–94	< 92

Table 20.3 Assessment of severity of asthma exacerbations in children.

of a severe condition, 92–94% of moderate and > 94% of a mild attack.

Lung function. As the best measurement of airway obstruction, *PEF should be measured whenever possible* in children ≥ 5 years. However, in the acute situation, it may be better to treat the child than to use the time training him/her in lung function measurements. The forced expiratory manoeuvres will increase bronchoconstriction.

High-risk patients. It is common to underestimate the severity of the condition in *infants*, who generally are more severely obstructed than older children and are at increased risk. Other characteristics of high-risk patients are: recent withdrawal of *oral steroid, hospitalization* for asthma in past year, earlier *catastrophic attack*, psychosocial problems and poor compliance.

Beta₂ agonists. An inhaled beta₂ agonist is superior to treatment with other bronchodilators by other routes. In contrast to common belief, infants do have bronchial beta₂ receptors and respond to beta₂ agonists (terbutaline and salbutamol).

Nebulizers *are the delivery system of choice in the treatment of acute severe asthma in all age groups of hospitalized children,* even though, in school children, the same results can be obtained with other inhalation systems. The dose depends upon the nebulizer brand and the volume fill. *High doses* are more effective than low doses, and *continuous nebulization* produces better results than the same dose nebulized intermittently, but this treatment will result in systemic side-effects.

Spacers require lower doses than nebulizers to produce the same response. Frequent administration from a spacer of a beta₂ agonist is highly efficient.

DPIs *should not be used for acute asthma in children ≤5 years,* as they may not be able to generate a sufficient inspiratory flow rate.

MDIs. The same is true for *conventional MDIs,* which are used only when another delivery system is not available.

Systemic administration. An *intravenous loading dose* is followed by a *continuous infusion.* Standard doses are not suitable for optimal therapy, as there is a *considerable inter-individual variation. Dosing should be individualized* under the monitoring of the therapeutic response and the occurrence of side-effects. For *subcutaneous or intramuscular injection,* salbutamol or terbutaline are preferable to adrenaline, which causes more side-effects.

Side-effects. Generally treatment of children with beta₂ agonists is *very safe.* Nebulized and systemic administration causes side-effects but they are not serious. Skeletal muscle *tremor,* *palpitations* and some agitation are the most common complaints. As in adults, there is an *increase in pulse rate* and a *fall in plasma potassium*.

Corticosteroids. Systemic steroids are beneficial in the management of acute severe asthma. Usually the drug is given orally but intravenous administration is necessary in very severe cases. If oral treatment is started early during an exacerbation, for example due to a viral airway infection, it may prevent the development of acute severe asthma, and perhaps inhaled steroids can do the same.

Theophylline has been used frequently for acute asthma in children but the documentation is not convincing, and *its role in acute asthma can be questioned*. Theophylline *can add little* to the effect of frequent inhalations of beta$_2$ agonists. Its *side-effects are numerous* (anorexia, nausea, vomiting, headache, CNS stimulation, tachycardia, arrhythmias, abdominal pain, diarrhoea, gastric bleeding, seizures, death). An intravenous bolus of 6 mg/kg lean body weight can be given to children who are not on oral theophylline. Continued theophylline infusion must be calculated precisely and plasma levels measured.

Ipratropium bromide delivered from a nebulizer may have a role as an adjunct to inhaled beta$_2$ agonists in the treatment of acute asthma, as the combined treatment produces slightly better results than the beta$_2$ agonist alone.

Management outside hospital. A child with acute asthma should be seen without delay. A *beta$_2$ agonist* is administered preferably *by a MDI with a spacer*. Give one puff every minute until satisfactory improvement occurs, that is, the clinical condition is changed into mild severity (Table 20.3). If inhaled treatment cannot be given terbutaline or salbutamol can be administered subcutaneously or intramuscularly.

Following a *mild attack inhaled steroid* is added until the condition has been stable for one week. Following a *moderate attack* a short course of prednisolone is also given. A child with a *severe attack* is admitted to hospital without delay.

Hospital management. In hospital the initial treatment consists of *inhaled beta₂ agonist* from an *oxygen-driven nebulizer*, followed by oral *prednisolone*, or in the critically ill child, intravenous methylprednisolone (Table 20.4). When the response to initial treatment is poor *nebulized ipratropium bromide* and *intravenous beta₂ agonist* (or theophylline) can be added.

Antibiotics are only given to patients with bacterial infections. Cough medicine is useless. *Sedatives are dangerous* and may induce respiratory failure and apnoea.

Intensive care and assisted ventilation. Children with acute severe asthma require intensive monitoring by experienced staff and all patients with life-threatening features (Table 20.5) not responding convincingly to treatment require intensive care.

Drug dosing in acute childhood asthma	
Beta₂ agonists	
Nebulizer	Salbutamol 0.2 mg/kg or terbutaline 0.4 mg/kg (max 5 mg in preschool children and 7.5 mg in school children). May be repeated at frequent intervals
Spacer or other inhaler	One puff every minute until satisfactory response Maximum dose: salbutamol 50 μg or terbutaline 100 μg/kg
Subcutaneous or intramuscular	Salbutamol or terbutaline 10 μg/kg
Intravenous	Loading dose: salbutamol/terbutaline 2–5 μg/kg Continuous: salbutamol/terbutaline 5 μg/kg/h
Corticosteroids	
Oral prednisolone	Loading dose: 1–2 mg/kg (max 60 mg) Continuous: 2 mg/kg/day divided into 2 doses
Intravenous methyl-prednisolone	Loading dose: 1–2 mg/kg Continuous: 1 mg/kg 6 hourly
Intravenous hydrocortisone	Loading dose: 10 mg/kg Continuous: 5 mg/kg 6 hourly

Table 20.4 Recommended average doses of the various drugs used to treat acute severe asthma in all age groups of children.

Life-threatening features
PEF < 40% of best
Cyanosis
Bradycardia
Fatigue/exhaustion
Reduced consciousness
Silent chest
Paradoxical thoraco-abdominal movement
Disappearance of retractions without concomitant clinical improvement

Table 20.5 Life-threatening features in childhood asthma requiring urgent anaesthesiological assistance.

Assisted ventilation is started when indicated by the clinical condition and repeated blood gas measurements.

Recovery, discharge, prevention. *High-dose inhaled steroid* is introduced as early as possible in order to make the *prednisolone* treatment period as short as possible. It is usually 1–2 weeks, while the inhaled steroid should continue for at least 4–8 weeks, because the child after recovery remains vulnerable with hyper-responsive airways.

The patient is *discharged* when symptoms have disappeared and PEF is > 75% of personal best and diurnal variation of PEF is < 25%. If he/she is discharged too early, there is a 25% risk of relapse within a few weeks.

In order to prevent new episodes it is useful to *investigate the circumstances of admission*. All patients should have a written *self-management plan* informing them at what PEF values or level of symptoms they should increase their treatment, how treatment should be increased and for how long, and when to call the doctor, or remit themselves to hospital.

Chapter 21: Immunotherapy

Specific immunotherapy (hyposensitization) consists of a series of subcutaneous *injections of allergen extract* with the aim of reducing the patient's sensitivity to the allergen in question and with that the allergic *symptoms in the conjunctiva, nose and bronchi* (immunotherapy with venoms is discussed in Chapter 23).

Indications

A series of placebo controlled studies have shown efficacy of immunotherapy with *pollen, mite and animal* extracts. It is still an open question whether the therapy can alter the natural history of allergic diseases, and, therefore, it is difficult to give precise guidelines for the use of immunotherapy. Opinions vary about *when and how often* to start this treatment.

Prerequisites for therapy. The specific diagnosis must be correct and allergen exposure must be a major cause of symptoms. Treatment of a positive skin test of little importance to the patient's disease is futile.

Patient age. Immunotherapy is a treatment for *young adults and children*, aged 5 years and above. In the elderly, IgE-mediated reactions are less important, and the risk of serious side-effects is increased (concurrent cardiovascular disease).

Pollen allergy is the major indication for immunotherapy. Controlled studies have shown that therapy with *grass, ragweed, birch, mugwort, cedar and parietaria* has a clear effect on *rhino-conjunctivitis* and *asthma* symptoms.

Obviously a patient with mild pollen allergy and occasional rhino-conjunctivitis symptoms does not require immunotherapy, while it has a clear role in patients with severe symptoms not controlled by pharmacotherapy (Fig. 21.1). Not only the *severity of the symptoms* but also the *length of the pollen season* is of

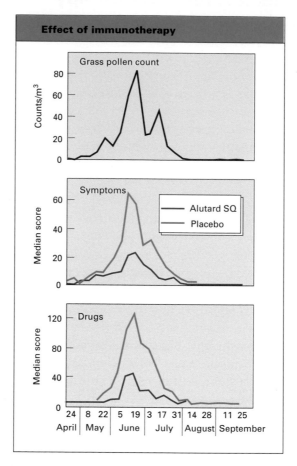

Fig. 21.1 Average weekly grass pollen count, and symptom and medication scores for allergen and placebo groups. (From Varney VA, Gaga M, Frew AJ, Aber VR, Kay AB, Durham SR. Usefulness of immunotherapy in patients with severe summer hay fever uncontrolled by anti-allergic drugs. *Br Med J*, 1991; 302: 265–9.)

importance. Thus, a long pollen season, a high degree of allergy and heavy pollen exposure all speak in favour of immunotherapy.

House dust mite. Studies have shown efficacy in children with mite allergy, while the results in adults are less impressive. Immunotherapy may be tried in children and youngsters who still have symptoms in spite of a mite avoidance programme.

Immunotherapy is not indicated in patients with severe asthma, or with a significant irreversible component ($FEV_1 < 70\%$), due to poor efficacy and risk of serious allergen-induced bronchoconstriction. Thus, the ideal patient for immunotherapy is a young person who suffers from *severe rhinitis* and *mild asthma*.

Animal proteins. Immunotherapy can have some effect in patients with allergy to mammals (demonstrated with cat allergen). It may be considered in selected cases when avoidance is not possible: (1) in *occupational allergies* (veterinarians, farmers, laboratory workers); and (2) in *highly allergic children* who cannot attend ordinary school education due to animal protein in schoolmates' clothes.

Immunotherapy should not be used instead of avoidance. It is a poor allergist who tells his patient that he can keep his pet while he is being 'cured' for his allergy by a series of injections. Immunotherapy can only reduce clinical sensitivity.

Contra-indications. Immunotherapy is a treatment for otherwise healthy young persons with good compliance to therapy. Abuse of alcohol or drugs, cardiovascular disease, use of beta-blockers, fixed airway obstruction and severe asthma are contra-indications, the latter because the expected benefit is small and the risk of serious reactions considerable.

Possible modes of action

The mechanism(s) by which immunotherapy exerts its beneficial effect is unclear. The therapy induces a series of immunological changes which may be responsible for symptom relief or epiphenomena (Fig. 21.2).

Technique and safety

Choice of allergen(s). It is advisable to *select one or two* allergens based on the result of allergy testing, knowledge of allergen occurrence in the patient's environment, and the possibilities of allergen avoidance.

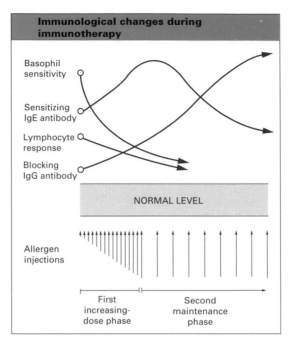

Fig. 21.2 Immunological changes during immunotherapy.

Allergen extracts. It is important always to use high-quality, *standardized allergen extracts* which have little batch-to-batch variation. *Aqueous extracts* have a short shelf-life, require many injections, and systemic reactions are relatively frequent. When extracts are physically modified by aluminium hydroxide or tyrosine, allergen absorption is delayed. Such *depot extracts* are usually preferred as they require fewer injections and the risk of systemic reactions is reduced.

Technique. Immunotherapy consists of two phases, the *increasing-dose phase* and the *maintenance phase*.

When a *depot preparation* is used, weekly injections are given in the first phase, and this interval is increased to 6–8 weeks in the second phase.

When an *aqueous extract* is used, the first phase can be completed within one week when it is given as a *rush regimen* in a hospitalized patient by administering 2–6 daily injections. An alternative is a *clustered regimen*, in which 2–4 injections are given in a day and repeated after 1–2 weeks.

Pollen immunotherapy can be given as *pre-seasonal* and as *perennial* therapy. Perennial therapy requires the lowest number of injections and is therefore preferable. The duration of therapy is usually *3–5 years*.

Choice of dose. During the increasing-dose phase the dose is doubled at each injection, but only when the preceding injection has not caused a large local or any systemic reaction.

The optimal maintenance dose is, in principle, the highest tolerated dose not eliciting side-effects. It is important for safety that the maintenance dose is given at regular intervals, following strict safety rules.

Precautions. Even a perfectly undertaken course of immunotherapy is associated with a risk of severe allergic reactions (anaphylactic shock, severe bronchoconstriction).

Therapy is only justified if all possible attempts are made to reduce this risk to zero. Most important is: (1) always to have adrenaline at hand; (2) always to have the patient wait for at least 30 minutes; (3) never to give an injection to a patient having an asthma episode; (4) to follow the recommendations in Malling H-J, Weeke B. EAACI immunotherapy position paper, *Allergy*, 1993; 48(suppl 14): 9–36.

Chapter 22: Anaphylaxis

An anaphylactic reaction (anaphylactic shock) is usually IgE mediated, but also other mechanisms can play a role (Table 22.1). The potency of all inducers of anaphylaxis is increased when they are given by the *parenteral route*, especially

Types of anaphylactic reactions
IgE-mediated reaction   Penicillin
Immune complex mediated reaction   Blood products
Direct effect on mast cells   Radiocontrast media
Abnormal arachidonic acid metabolism   Acetylsalicylic acid

Table 22.1 Types of anaphylactic reactions with examples of causative agents.

intravenously. The clinical consequence of an anaphylactic reaction is more severe in *asthma* patients and in patients on *beta-blockers*.

Causative agents

The list of agents, headed by drugs, is long, and only the most important are mentioned.

Drugs. The most frequent causes of anaphylaxis are *penicillin* and the synthetic penicillin derivatives. Other causes are heterologous antisera, peptide hormones, enzymes, radiographic contrast media, opiates, anaesthetics, muscle relaxants, pentamidine, plasma expanders, *acetylsalicylic acid* and other NSAIDs.

Foods. Almost any food may cause anaphylactic reactions but those most commonly responsible are *eggs, milk, nuts, fish* and *shellfish*.

Stinging insects. Venoms from stinging insects, especially of the *Hymenoptera* order, are relatively common causes of anaphylaxis (see Chapter 23).

Human products. *Blood, plasma* and *immunoglobulins* can cause anaphylactic reactions via immune complexes and complement activation. In the rare cases, *seminal fluid* has provoked IgE-mediated anaphylaxis during coitus.

Immunotherapy frequently results in slight systemic reactions but anaphylaxis is rare.

Latex. Recently, IgE-mediated allergy to latex has become a prominent cause of anaphylaxis in *medical personnel* and even in *patients* due to intra-operative exposure to the surgeons' gloves (see Chapter 24).

Physical stimuli. A patient with *cold-induced* urticaria can get an anaphylactic reaction if he jumps into cold water. *Physical exercise* can worsen an allergic reaction, for example to food, and in some cases only a combined exposure will result in anaphylaxis.

Idiopathic. In the rare case, anaphylaxis can occur repeatedly without any obvious reason.

Clinical presentation

The skin, upper and lower airways, cardiovascular system and gastro-intestinal tract may be affected singly or in combination. Death is due to suffocation (laryngeal ocdema, asthma) or cardiac arrest (hypotension, arrhythmias).

Initial symptoms. Symptoms may *start within minutes*, and the earlier they occur, the more severe the reaction. The first symptom is *pruritus*, followed by *erythema* and, in severe cases, *loss of consciousness*. The *pulse is rapid* and weak and the *blood pressure low*.

Skin symptoms. The initial pruritus and flushing may progress to include *urticaria* and *angioedema*.

Respiratory symptoms. Early stages of *laryngeal oedema* may be experienced as hoarseness, which is of grave importance as oedema can quickly progress to asphyxia. Severe bronchoconstriction may develop in patients with *asthma*.

Cardiovascular symptoms. Extravasation of fluid and vasodilatation can cause *hypotension and shock*. The circulatory collapse together with *hypoxaemia* predispose to *myocardial infarction*. The risk of death from anaphylaxis is considerably increased in the elderly and in patients with myocardial disease.

Differential diagnosis. Collapse after an injection can be due to anaphylaxis or a *vasovagal syncope*. In the latter the *pulse is slow*, there is *no pruritus* and *no skin or airway symptoms*, and the symptoms are immediately *relieved by recumbency*.

Treatment

Early recognition and prompt institution of therapy is of utmost importance (Table 22.2).

Adrenaline (epinephrine) is the *essential drug*. As soon as anaphylaxis is recognized, it is given *intramuscularly*, 0.5 mg (0.01 mg/kg body weight in children). As adrenaline has a short half-life, the injection can be *repeated* at 30 minute intervals. If

Treatment of anaphylaxis
Treatment in office
Have patient lie down and call for assistance
Inject intramuscularly 0.5 mg adrenaline
Insert an intravenous line
Give a number of inhalations from a beta$_2$ inhaler
If you have time, inject an H$_1$ antihistamine
If the patient is still hypotensive or does not have free airways make arrangements for transport to an intensive care unit
Treatment under transportation
Administer pure oxygen
Give intramuscularly 0.5 mg adrenaline every 20–30 minutes
If blood pressure is immeasurable, give 0.3 mg adrenaline intravenously (flush with saline)
If adequate ventilation cannot be maintained, insert an oral airway and ventilate with a compressible bag (oxygen)

Table 22.2 Treatment of anaphylaxis.

the condition is *life-threatening*, 0.3 mg adrenaline can be given *intravenously* (in a running drip or flush with saline).

Oxygen. *Early administration* of oxygen *for hypotension and airway obstruction* is important for the prevention of cardiac complications.

Intravenous fluid. Fully developed anaphylactic shock is associated with a considerable loss of intravascular fluid. An *intravenous line* is essential for fluid replacement therapy and is always necessary to ensure medication.

Free airways. *Upper airway oedema* can develop rapidly, requiring intubation or tracheotomy. When it is threatening, *adrenaline* is given in the highest tolerable dose, and the patient is placed in a *half-sitting position* with the neck extended. *Pure oxygen* is administered. In all *asthma* patients, a *beta$_2$ agonist* is administered early, preferably by the inhaled route.

Antihistamines and corticosteroids. An antihistamine is given, preferably intravenously, following the initial use of adrenaline. Steroids in status asthmaticus doses are indicated in severe cases to prevent a secondary relapse.

Prevention

The life-threatening nature of anaphylaxis makes prevention the keystone of therapy. Always *prefer the oral route* to the parenteral, and require a *clear indication for intravenous drug use*. Always *be prepared* to treat anaphylaxis and *have adrenaline at hand* whenever an injection is given.

Chapter 23: Allergy to bee and wasp

Stinging insects are responsible for a vast number of trivial skin reactions. Occasionally, however, the reactions can be dangerous and even fatal when individuals develop an allergic reaction to the venom.

Stinging insects belong to two super-families: (1) *honeybees,* which can be responsible for multiple stings when their hive is endangered, but are not aggressive away from their hive; (2) *wasp, yellow jacket and hornet,* which are aggressive and can sting, even when unprovoked. There is marked cross-reactivity between venoms from wasp, yellow jacket and hornet, but bee venom is different.

Local reactions. Pain, erythema and swelling, lasting for 1–2 days are a *normal reaction* to stings. A large local reaction can be due to allergy or infection.

Systemic reactions. A systemic reaction is always due to *allergy.* It can consist of urticaria, angioedema, asthma, anaphylaxis and cardiovascular collapse.

Natural history. Following a serious systemic reaction, 50% will get another serious reaction with a subsequent sting. The risk of death from anaphylaxis is relatively high in the elderly and very low in children.

Diagnosis. The diagnosis is generally self-evident, but problems arise in the identification of the insect. The honeybee is readily identifiable because it leaves its sting in place. *Allergy testing* is only carried out in patients with *systemic reactions.* A *skin-prick test* is the most rapid and economic method, but RAST is a good and safe substitute or additive.

Management of acute reactions. The sting is removed when possible. Relief of local symptoms can be obtained by pressing an *ice cube* against the sting site.

Itching, urticaria and mild cases are treated with an *oral antihistamine*. A severe, generalized reaction is treated with *adrenaline* following the general rules for treatment of anaphylaxis (see Chapter 22). Upper airway obstruction often plays an important role in venom allergy.

A patient who has had a severe generalized reaction should carry an *emergency-kit*, consisting of a pre-loaded syringe with adrenaline and an antihistamine tablet.

Venom immunotherapy is offered to adult patients who have had a *generalized reaction with respiratory or cardiovascular symptoms* and show a *positive skin test or RAST*. Children are usually not treated because fatalities are almost unknown in childhood (Table 23.1). Immunotherapy should not be used in patients on *beta-blocker* therapy, and it should not be started during *pregnancy*.

The goal for therapy is a maintenance dose of *100 µg venom protein*, the equivalent of a few stings, which gives a 90% protection rate. The duration of venom immunotherapy is *3–5 years*.

Indication for venom immunotherapy	
Patients	**Indication**
Adults with a severe systemic reaction (respiratory or cardiovascular involvement)	yes
Adults with a moderate systemic reaction (urticaria, angioedema, mild asthma)	no/yes*
Adults with a mild systemic reaction	no
Children with a systemic reaction	no
Patients with a large local reaction	no

Table 23.1 Indication for immunotherapy of patients with reactions to insect stings and a clear-cut positive allergy test. * Depends on frequency of reaction, likelihood of future exposure and access to medical service.

Chapter 24: Latex allergy

It has long been known that rubber gloves can cause *contact eczema* by a *Type IV reaction* to *chemical additives* to rubber. This delayed-type reaction can be diagnosed by *patch-testing* and will not be discussed further. More recently, an IgE-mediated *Type I reaction*, or immediate-type reaction, to *latex protein* was described as an *important cause of occupational allergy* among health care personnel.

Allergens

Latex is the milky sap collected by tapping the rubber tree.
Rubber is a widespread product and the variety of articles containing latex is considerable. The most important are *gloves, medical equipment (catheters, tubes),* condoms and balloons. Latex allergens show *cross-reactivity* with some fruit allergens (banana, avocado, kiwi).

Risk factors

An *atopic background* and *hand eczema* predispose to latex allergy. Due to the dramatic rise in the use of gloves, 10–20% of *dental workers* and *nurses* working in operating units are now allergic. Patients who undergo multiple operations or are chronically exposed to latex medical devices (catheters) are at risk, especially *children with spina bifida* or severe urogenital defects.

Clinical manifestations

Contact urticaria of the back of the hands and fingers, which arises within minutes of direct contact with gloves, is a good indicator of latex allergy.

Cornstarch powder, which absorbs latex proteins in gloves, becomes airborne and can induce *symptoms in eyes, nose and bronchi* within minutes after a package of gloves is opened.

Anaphylactic reactions predominantly occur during intra-abdominal surgery, due to contact with the surgeon's gloves, but can occur following tracheal intubation, insertion of a catheter, gynaecologic examination and barium enema examination, as the rectal catheter has a latex cuff.

Diagnosis

Skin-prick testing is an easy, specific and sensitive way to diagnose latex allergy but extracts are not yet standardized. At present, skin-testing is more sensitive than *in vitro* testing. *Provocation testing* consists of wearing a latex glove and of handling boxes containing gloves.

Prevention

People with a history of *atopic disease and eczema* are advised to use synthetic non-latex gloves. In *children with spina bifida* latex products should be avoided completely. *Washing the gloves* is a poor second best. Stringent elimination of latex from the operating room is needed to protect a sensitive patient.

Index